THE INFERTILE
COUPLE AND MODERN
COST-EFFECTIVE
MANAGEMENT

THE INFERTILE COUPLE AND MODERN COST-EFFECTIVE MANAGEMENT

WITH SPECIAL EMPHASIS FOR RESOURCE-POOR DEVELOPING COUNTRIES

DR. NORBERT I. EKEH MD

To order additional copies of this book, contact:
Xlibris Corporation
1-888-795-4274
www.Xlibris.com
Orders@Xlibris.com
88323

CONTENTS

Foreword

This concise, well-illustrated, and well-referenced textbook written by Dr. Norbert I. Ekeh MD has provided a comprehensive and an up-to-date modern infertility management not only for all health care practitioners in the field but also for the couple and clients who are keen to learn all they could about their condition as well as health care administrators.

The list of abbreviations at the beginning of the book as well as the glossary/definitions at the end would help those with minimal medical terminologies understand and enjoy their read of the text. The chapter on potential effective and low-cost ART for resource-poor countries is a challenge even for us in the so-called developed economies. The ethical dimensions, especially the Catholic objection to modern IVF treatment, are not treated lightly. All facets of modern infertility treatment are expertly treated and referenced from timed intercourse to more complex and modern issues such as surrogacy, acupuncture, and medical tourism in infertility treatment.

Having worked closely with Dr. Ekeh in this exciting field of modern infertility management for over ten years now, I confess that this book is a must read for all in the field, clinicians and clients alike. I would also dare recommend it for all health care planners, especially those in resource-poor countries.

A. Fenton, MS, RT
Programs Director,
MCF Reproductive & Health Services Ltd
Toronto, Canada.

Preface

The idea for this book is borne out of a combination of observations and events happening in my life over the past few years. It all started with a casual observation during one of my visits to my home country, Nigeria, of an apparent 'explosion' in infertile couples seeking 'divine intervention' to their problems. It also occurred to me that while my parents' generation often appeared to have had an average of six to 7 children, my own generation seems to be whittled down to only about three children per family but most importantly, there are many couples seemingly unable to have any child. I then decided to do something about this by a firm decision to return to Nigeria to practice solely as a fertility specialist. I resigned my job as an Obstetrician/ Gynaecologist to concentrate on infertility while studying for a masters' degree course in Clinical Embryology on a part time basis from the University of Leeds, UK. While doing my research project for this master's degree, I chose to pursue my interest at the provision of cheap and effective Assisted Reproductive Technology (ART) treatments in modern infertility management including potential cheap alternatives. With the successful completion of my research project, this is an attempt at putting down in a book all available modern effective infertility treatment strategies in terms of low-tech and high-tech fertility treatments as well as potential low-cost and effective treatment strategies detailed in chapter 5, some of which are not yet clinically applicable. It is hoped that this book will help stimulate research in some of these innovative approach for the benefit of all including the infertile in resource-poor countries.

Acknowledgments

I wish to express my deep appreciation of the encouragements by my lecturers at the University of Leeds for all their encouragements during my MSc research project, which kick-started this book. My special thanks go to my head of department, Professor Helen Picton, as well as doctors David Miller and John Huntriss for all their support during my project that metamorphosed into this book.

I wish also to acknowledge the best efforts of fertility clinicians including gynecologists, embryologists, and all who practice assisted reproductive techniques (ART) in resource-poor countries of the world. The challenge is the provision of the effective modern ART in the context of poor infrastructure (especially electricity and water) and at an affordable price!

Finally, I wish to thank God almighty for enabling me to father my two extremely intelligent and lovely children, Odera and Nwadi.

List of Abbreviations

AH   assisted hatching

AI   artificial insemination

AMH   anti-Müllerian hormone

ART   advanced reproductive technology

ASRM   American Society for Reproductive Medicine

BCP   birth control pills

CC   clomiphene citrate

CCCT   clomiphene citrate challenge test

CO2   carbon dioxide

CASA   computer-assisted semen analysis

DI   donor sperm insemination

DHEA   dehydroepiandrosterone

DNA   deoxyribonucleic acid

E2   estradiol

ER   egg retrieval

ESHRE   European Society for Human Reproduction and Embryology

ET	embryo transfer
FET	frozen embryo transfers
FSH	follicle-stimulating hormone
FSP	fallopian tube sperm perfusion
GA	general anesthesia
GH	growth hormone
Gn	gonadotropin
GnRH-a	gonadotropin-releasing hormone agonist
GnRH-A	gonadotropin-releasing hormone antagonist
High Tech	high technologically intensive
hMG	human menopausal gonadotropin
HSG	hysterosalpingogram
Hx	history
ICI	intracervical insemination
ICSI	intracytoplasmic sperm injection
ICU	intensive care unit
IFI	intrafallopian insemination
ITI	intratubal insemination
IUC	intrauterine culture
IUI	intrauterine insemination
IUTP	intrauterine tuboperitoneal insemination

IVC	intravaginal culture
IVF	in vitro fertilization
IVI	intravaginal insemination
IUL	intrauterine life
IVM	in vitro maturation
LH	luteinizing hormone
Low Tech	low technologically intensive
LPD	luteal phase defect
MAR test	mixed antiglobulin reaction test
MESA	microscopic epididymal sperm aspiration
NSAIDs	nonsteroidal anti-inflammatory drugs
OATS	oligoasthenoteratozoospermia
OHSS	ovarian hyperstimulation syndrome
PCT	postcoital test
PE	physical examination
PESA	percutaneous epididymal sperm aspiration
PGD	preimplantation genetic diagnosis
PG	prostaglandin
PID	pelvic inflammatory disease
POF	premature ovarian failure
PZD	partial zona dissection

RBC	red blood cells
ROS	reactive oxygen species
Rx	treatment
SA	semen analysis
SIFT	sperm intrafallopian transfer
SLE	systemic lupus erythematosus
Sono HSG	sonographic hysterosalpingogram
STD	sexually transmitted disease
SZI	subzonal sperm injection
TB	tuberculosis
TESA	testicular sperm aspiration
TESE	testicular sperm extraction
US	ultrasound
USA	United States of America
WBC	white blood cells or leukocytes
WHO	World Health Organization
ZP	zona pellucida

Introduction

When Rachel saw that she was not bearing Jacob any children, she became jealous of her sister. So she said to Jacob, "Give me children, or I'll die!"

The Holy Bible-Genesis 30:1

I feel very confused, afraid and have lots of unanswered questions. . . . 'I felt terrible and alone . . . . with guilt and shame wondering why me? . . . . what have I done to deserve this . . . . I developed low self esteem wondering whether my husband, friends and family would accept me . . . . . or divorce me . . . . at same time, I am easily irritated and angry, even at listening to well-intentioned advice . . . .

The infertile

As the above quotes indicate, the personal devastation and distress experienced by individuals and couples with inability to establish a desired family unit has been documented in all cultures since the beginning of recorded time (Parnell T, 2005). In recent times, the USA Supreme Court in affirming lower court decisions of infertility being a disability defined the ability to conceive as a basic life activity (Gleicher N, 1998). But this disability and personal tragedy being experienced all over the world are further compounded for the infertile women in the resource-poor developing countries like Nigeria where these women have been documented with a far reaching continuum of consequences ranging from blame, guilt, fear, social isolation/alienation, increased violence, divorce, polygamy to even murder being perpetrated on them; also there is increased exposure to multiple sexual partners and STDs as well as helplessness, economic destitution and suicide on their own (Araoye MO, 2003; Boerma JT et al, 2001). And implications have been extrapolated for neonatal and maternal morbidity/ mortality (Joffe M et al, 1994, Basso O et al, 2003; Basso O et al, 2005).

Furthermore, motherhood in the developing nations is often perceived as a way to enhance the woman's status within the family unit and unto the wider community at large. As such, these women are often willing to undertake whatever it takes to achieve motherhood. But proven modern fertility care and treatments are either not readily available, accessible and/or expensive and therefore not within reach for most of these women who are then driven to consult alternative traditional or faith-based healers, using traditional herbs and/or beliefs some of which could be very bizarre such as being 'bewitched' by jealous neighbours, co-wives or mother-in laws, being 'possessed' by evil spirits or bad ancestral spirits, etc!

There are also harsh economic realities with respect to infertility in developing countries. In the absence of social security provisions as in most developed economies and without their own children, many men and women may starve to death especially in their old age! In some communities, the infertile are perceived to be the source of evil in the community and then ostracized or made objects of shame and humiliation and, or denying them proper burial rites, etc.

Therefore, infertility in resource-poor developing countries of the world poses a myriad of complex and rather unique problems far and above those well documented for the developed nations by rather being transformed from an acute, private agonizing condition as usually observed in most developed nations into a harsh, public stigmatised condition with the continuum of evolving complex and devastating consequences alluded to above.

The WHO has earlier defined health as 'a state of complete physical, mental and social well-being, and not merely the absence of disease or infirmity' By this definition, infertility is therefore, a disease condition. And in fact, it could be argued that fewer disease conditions could wreck as much profound and pervasive effects on individuals' and families' well-being as a whole than infertility. In this regards, infertility has been compared to cancer!

But some have argued that over-population should rather be the major issue facing most of the resource-poor developing countries such that family planning and contraception should be the main focus rather than infertility management. Others further argued that these countries with poor resources and infrastructure are saturated with high prevalence of many communicable and preventable diseases such as tuberculosis, malaria, HIV/AIDS, typhoid disease, diarrhoeal infectious diseases, helminthiasis, etc. All theses arguments are simply not tenable. Take for instance the HIV/AIDS. If it justifiable to provide the very expensive medication cocktail needed to treat such a condition in these poor countries which then prolong the lives of all those treated, would this also not have on 'over-population' effect by enabling more people living with this condition rather than having died with full blown AIDS? As such, why would treating infertility, even with the expensive ART equipments not be reasonable justified in these poor resource countries? Some reason that the aged-old dictum, "prevention is always better than cure" should be the goal rather treating the infertile. Of course so is with all known ailments including the densely prevalent communicable diseases already mentioned above! Ideally and if possible, all diseases and illnesses should rather be prevented such that there would not be any need to treat. Unfortunately this is not only feasible but also impossible to achieve medically as there would always be the need to treat diseases. Some others have gone further narrowing their arguments only against the introduction of modern effective but expensive infertility treatments currently widely available in developed countries (Okonofua FE, 1996), although with recent successful application of these treatment options in some private infertility clinics/ hospitals in Nigeria, the arguments seem to be waning in favour of these new private initiatives (Okonofua FE, 2003). Still some argue that adoption should be the norm for the infertile considering the numerous poor and, or orphaned children in resource-poor developing countries but again, this is not feasible practically. Moreover, anecdotal evidence indicates that there are still many cultural biases against adoption in most developing countries.

Therefore, the idea that modern infertility treatments including the expensive ART which has been established to be very effective in the modern management of the 'few' with infertility should not be a health priority in resource poor countries is based on the above fallacious assumptions while at same time, there is the utter disregard of the devastating and potential life-threatening consequences already outlined above.

It is also important to highlight that tubal diseases is the underlying cause of most cases of female infertility seen in consultation in sub Sahara Africa. This is in contradistinction to tubal causes seen in the more affluent developed countries (35% v 85% in Africa; Gates W et al, 1985). It then stands to reason that every effort should be made to make IVF (the main core ART, which was originally conceptualized to by-pass tubal diseases) as widely available as possible to the infertile in these resource-poor countries rather than the current very limited access when compared to the developed nations.

This book aims to provide a unique perspective on modern and effective infertility management for all healthcare providers who may come in contact with the infertile couples, the patients themselves as well health policy administrators especially all those in resource-poor countries of the world. It is my firm belief that a diagnosis of infertility in today's world should not be synonymous with childlessness for any couple irrespective of their country of residence or their financial capability because the currently available modern infertility treatments offer a good rate of success. The challenge therefore, is provision of these modern effective treatments at an affordable cost to all i.e., cost-effective modern infertility treatments to all, irrespective of the couple's location in this wide world! The need for cheap ART or effective alternatives cannot therefore be over-emphasized. The race is on!

Chapter 1

BACKGROUND ON HUMAN
FERTILITY AND INFERTILITY

I simply assumed I was fertile, often taking measures to avoid getting pregnant . . . It now seems ironic that I cannot conceive now.

THE INFERTILE

Most couples simply assume, albeit naively, that they are fertile, expecting to conceive the first month they try. Fortunately, for some (as few as about 25% of cases), this is the case! The explanation is varied, but by far, the main reason is simply that we humans are not inherently designed to produce numerous babies either at once or in quick successions compared to other mammals like rabbits! Thus, even for a normal and very fertile couple having sexual intercourse regularly, their chance for achieving pregnancy in one cycle is at most 25%, but cumulatively and over a twelve-month period, this chance increases to between 80 and 90%. This has been defined in terms of fecundity and fecundability, that is, fertility potential in a single menstrual cycle. *Fecundity* is the probability of achieving a life birth via a single cycle while *fecundability* is the probability of achieving pregnancy in one cycle.

Based on the above, there is therefore the one in six couples in whom getting pregnant or achieving a life birth is no easy task, being labelled infertile, with the road ahead being rather long, tortuous, and rocky with consequent great toll on the couple's time, energy, emotions, finances, etc.

WHO had, in 1990, defined *infertility* as two years' exposure to pregnancy without conceiving, but a more widely applied clinical definition is failure of conception after twelve months of unprotected sexual intercourse. The time lag in this definition takes into cognizance the concept of the trying time in fecundity and fecundability! Another

1

slight modification is the addition of miscarriages or infertility to the definition such that infertility is now defined as the failure to conceive after twelve months of regular, unprotected sexual intercourse or the occurrence of more than two consecutive miscarriages or stillbirths (Greenhall E et al, 1990).

EPIDEMIOLOGY

Notwithstanding the time frame in the definition of infertility above, infertility from the epidemiological point of view is a very complex medical disorder with interplay of significant medical, psychosocial, cultural, and economic aspects.

PREVALENCE

The prevalence of infertility has been put at between 8 and 12% of couples all over the world (Reproductive Health Outlook 1997-2005). Prevalence has been reported to be higher in resource-poor developing countries compared to the developed countries (Lunenfielf B et al, 2004). In some developing countries, this figure could be as high as 30% (WHO 1991). In sub-Saharan Africa, an area dogged the "infertility belt," has one-third of all couples unable to reproduce during their reproductive lives (Cates et al. 1985). In Nigeria, infertility was found to be the leading reason for gynecological consultation (Okonofua FE, 1996) with a prevalence rate in about one-third of the couples (WHO 1991; Okonufua F, 1999). In 2002, the WHO estimated 186 million married women to be infertile all over the world, excluding China (Rutestain S et al, DHS Comparative Report no. 9).

WHO has been at the forefront of conducting epidemiological studies in infertility in resource-poor countries and producing recommendations (WHO 2002). This WHO 2002 document not only suggested a focus on preventive strategies but also recommended the collection, collation, and interpretation of population-derived data and provision of guidelines with culturally sensitive biases.

AGE AND FERTILITY

Natural fertility declines with age. This is especially applicable to the human female species, where the optimum time for them to conceive is in their late teens and early twenties. Meantime to conception (i.e., time at which 50% of women conceive) increases with age from four months in normal "fertile" women younger than thirty to nine months in similar women older than thirty-five (Van Noord-Zaastra BM et al, 1991).

The graph below is from the 2006 ART success rates report data from the Centers for Disease Control (CDC), Atlanta, USA. The graph clearly illustrates the effect age has on fertility, especially when the success rate with donor eggs was superimposed, revealing no drop in pregnancy rate!

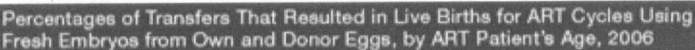

Percentages of Transfers That Resulted in Live Births for ART Cycles Using Fresh Embryos from Own and Donor Eggs, by ART Patient's Age, 2006

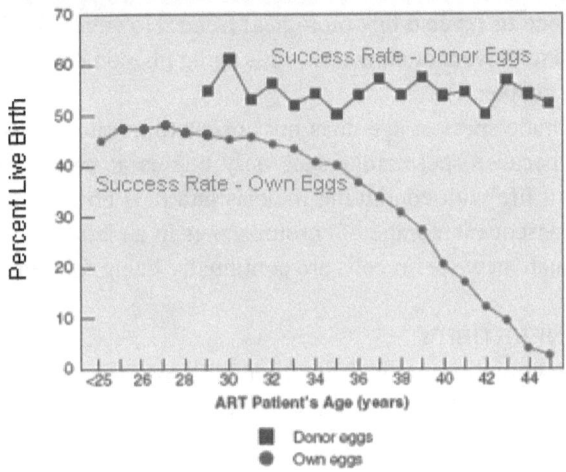

A classic 1950s large-population epidemiological study in noncontraceptive-using homogenous religious sect in the Dakota and Montana areas of USA (Tietze C, 1957) provides the most fertile group ever studied; that is, only about 2.4% of the women were childless. Yet analysis of the relationship between female age and fertility found the following correlation:

- By age thirty, 7% of couples were infertile.
- By age thirty-five, 11% of couples were infertile.
- By age forty, 33% of couples were infertile.
- By age forty-five, 87% of couples were infertile!

In terms of ovarian reserve, a typical woman has 12% of her reserve by age thirty and only about 3% at age forty with 81% of variations in ovarian reserve being due to age alone (Wallace WHB et al, 2010). Furthermore, the incidence of spontaneous abortion is almost doubled in women in their late thirties, compared to women younger than thirty (Warburton D et al, 1986).

All these mentioned above combine to make age the single most important factor in female fertility!

The reasons why age affects primarily the females could be traced to the fact that their oocytes all enter the prophase 1 of meiosis, forming the primary oocytes between the twelfth and twenty-fifth week of intrauterine life and becoming arrested at the dictyotene stage of this prophase. Thus, the later in life from puberty to menopause whenever these oocytes are recruited, they had been frozen for a varying length of time in this relatively stable state of prophase 1 of meiosis but still with some potential for chromosomal or spindle damage and thus result to failure to either establish a pregnancy or to miscarry

3

or to then develop chromosomally abnormal babies. And because this is primarily a problem related to the chromosomes and cellular machinery of the eggs, there is so far little that can be done to reverse this biological trend. However, the search is on for treatment protocols to prevent or slow down this aging phenomenon (see treatment for poor responders in chapter 4).

In the human male species, age does not appear to be such a major factor as in females probably because spermatogenesis only begins at puberty and appears to continue throughout life with continuing meiosis and thus no arrests during meiotic cell division and consequent storage of chromosomes in an inherently unstable status as in females. As such, new sperm cells are continually being formed.

ETIOLOGY OF INFERTILITY

Infertility is a complex medical disorder with significant psychological and economical dimensions. It is also a unique medical condition in that it involves the couple rather than the individual male or female. However, and in most cases, the cause could be traced to either of the gender, being then classified as either male factor infertility or female factor infertility or sometimes to a combination of both. A WHO study of 5,800 infertile couples seeking help at thirty-three medical centers in both developed and developing countries found female causes accounted for 25-27% of infertility worldwide (with larger proportions accounted for by sub-Saharan Africa and Asia); male factors accounted for 8-22%, and combined male/female causes accounted for 21-38% (Gates W et al, 1985). For simplicity sake, the overall causes of infertility could be summarized thus:

- Male factor infertility 35%
- Female factor infertility 35%
- Combination of male and female factor 20%
- Unexplained 10%

I. Female Factor Infertility

Female infertility is also classified in terms of primary (no prior conception) or secondary (prior conception). The above-quoted WHO multinational study also displays regional variations with developing countries appearing to have a preponderance of secondary infertility (64% of infertile women in sub-Saharan Africa had diagnoses attributable to infection, about double the rate for other regions). At the core of the above classification are about 5% cases of all the infertile attributable to anatomical, endocrinological, genetic, and immunological problems (WHO, 1991).

Most classical texts often describe the causes of female infertility in terms of these categories:

1. General factors
    Age(probably the single most important factor
        for female infertility (see above))
    Smoking
    STDs
    Body weight and eating disorders

    Others (e.g., medical diseases including autoimmune diseases (SLE,
    autoimmune adrenalitis, etc.), alcohol and drugs, environmental and
    occupational factors—including stress, exercise excess, malnutrition, etc.)

2. Structural factors
    Hypothalamo-pituitary factors (e.g., hypogonadotropic anovulation)
    Ovarian factors (e.g., PCOS, premature ovarian
        failure (POF), luteal phase defects (LPD))
    Tuboperitoneal factors (e.g., endometriosis,
        PID, STDs, pelvic adhesions)
    Uterine factors (e.g., submucous fibroids, uterine synechia
        and adhesions (Asherman's syndrome), congenital
        uterine anomalies (septate, bicornuate, etc.))
    Cervical factors (e.g., cervical stenosis and blockage)
    Vulvovaginal factors (e.g., vaginal atresia)
3. Note that iatrogenic (surgical) removal and/or diseased destruction or damage
    of any of the above structures would impair fertility.
4. Genetic factors
    Turner's syndrome (X0 syndrome)
    Testicular feminization syndrome
    Trisomy X
    Gonadal dysgenesis
    Kallman's syndrome
    Cystic fibrosis
5. Unexplained

From an epidemiological viewpoint, female infertility could be classified in terms
of whether preventable or nonpreventable. This is especially significant for female
infertility viewed from the poor developing countries. The 5% cases of infertility quoted
in the WHO study above are essentially the nonpreventable causes and do not appear to
vary much across countries and regions of the world. Thus, and by far, the majority of the
infertility causes are potentially preventable, and it is these that are largely responsible
for intra/inter-regional variations in etiology all over the world and include these:

A. Infectious and parasitic disease

Especially the STDs, endometritis, and PID, including postabortal and postpartum; TB; schistosomiasis; malaria; etc.

STD/PID has been documented to be the leading preventable cause of infertility and, together with postpartum/postabortion infections, are of high prevalence in sub-Saharan Africa. Other rarer reproductive infections and parasitic diseases that could cause infertility include genital TB and schistosomiasis.

The risk of tubal-factor infertility increases with successive episodes of PID, thus: one episode 8% risk two episodes 22% risk three or more episodes 41% (STD, 1994)

B. Other diseases, including sickle-cell disease

C. Cultural practices, including genital mutilations and postpartum endometritis

Certain cultural practices, especially polygamy, which, instead of increasing fertility, has actually been demonstrated to be associated with infertility (Population Report Series 1983). Many explanations are given to explain this surprise finding, including the fact that the infertility in itself is often the cause of the polygamy without taking cognizance the fact of high male factor contribution to infertility. Female circumcision with associated genital mutilation could result in scarring and infections. Postpartum abstinence could lead to a husband having extramarital sex and contracting STD.

D. Environmental and dietary hazards

The reproductive systems of both the male and female are particularly vulnerable to the effects of the environment. Agricultural and industrial pollutants, including pesticides, could severely affect reproductive health. The semen of some infertile Nigerian men contains high levels of metabolites of a fungus called aflatoxins, known to infest many stable foods in tropical countries (Ibeh IN et al, 1994). Dietary habits—including excessive intake of alcohol, tobacco, caffeine—are also common.

E. Health care practices and policies

Certain health care practices and policies may affect fertility. Unhygienic delivery practices still prevalent in many developing countries lead to increased risks of postpartum abortions. Wide prevalence of "quack" practitioners of abortions leads to increased postabortion sepsis and various injuries to the reproductive tract. Even the practice of surgical hernia repairs by inexperienced surgeons had been reported to lead to increased risks of male infertility in Nigerian men due to vascular injuries (Kuku SF et al, 1989).

II. Male Factor Infertility

While women are oftentimes the focus of infertility management, research, and social blame, male factors are the cause or contributing factor in approximately half of infertile couples. Yet there has remained continuing difficulties in the diagnosis of male factor infertility. The WHO has since 1980 promoted and published diagnostic criteria based on conventional semen analyses, the most recent edition being the fifth in 2010. A few other studies have attempted functional rather than descriptive diagnostic criteria used by WHO (Hull MGR et al, 1985), but no matter the criteria used, male factor infertility has remained the commonest single diagnostic category for all-cause classification (Schmidt L et al, 1995).

The etiology of male factor infertility is commonly subdivided into obstructive and non-obstructive azoospermia, viewed as either defects with respect to sperm production or sperm delivery, although by far, the majority remain idiopathic as presented below:

A.   Idiopathic (40-50%)

B.   Obstructive azoospermia or altered transport (10-20%)
Erectile dysfunction
Retrograde ejaculation or other dysfunction
Hypospadias
Vas deferens absence (e.g., cystic fibrosis)
Epididymis absence

C.   Nonobstructive azoospermia
1.   Primary hypogonadism: testicular failure (30-40%)
Varicocele (40%)
Drugs and medications (gonadotoxins), including alcohol abuse
Testicular injuries and surgeries
Genital irradiation or chemotherapy
Testicular infection
Postpubertal mumps
STDs
Chromosomal abnormalities (e.g., Klinefelter's syndrome)
Exposures
To excess heat (hot tubs, saunas, prolonged
cycling or horse riding, etc.)
To toxic chemicals/gonadotoxins
To environmental pollutants and pesticides,
including cigarette smoke, etc.

2. Secondary hypogonadism: hypothalamo-pituitary testicular axis (2%)
   Hypogonadotropic hypogonadism
   Androgen excess (e.g., anabolic steroids)
   Estrogen excess (e.g., tumors)
   Pituitary tumors (e.g., adenomas)
   Infiltrative disorders (e.g., TB, sarcoidosis)

Note that a simple criterion for distinguishing between the obstructive and non-obstructive causes is via serum FSH level and testicular US.

Also, and from the above, it could be seen that male infertility lies at the crossroads between genetic determinants and environmental effects, being associated with a host of disease conditions, including testicular cancer (Hotaling et al, 2009).

Chapter 2

BASIC ANATOMY AND PHYSIOLOGY OF HUMAN REPRODUCTION

And God said unto them, be fruitful, and multiply, and replenish the earth.

—Genesis 1:28, the Holy Bible

This chapter is of vital importance in that it would aid the understanding of the complex processes involved in reproduction. Especially, it would aid clear understanding of timing of sexual intercourse to achieve pregnancy and why and how we perform insemination during ART and other ART procedures.

Reproduction, a process by which organisms create offspring, is one of the unique characteristics of living organisms. Human reproduction is an example of sexual reproduction whereby fertilization takes place inside the female body by act of copulation by male and female reproductive cells being brought in close proximity with resultant internal fertilization, gestation, and childbirth by the female reproductive system specially designed for this purpose. All these involve an integrated action of hormones, the nervous system, and the reproductive system. In recent times, artificial insemination may bypass the act of copulation.

Human reproductive systems are divided into internal reproductive organs and the external genitalia.

The internal reproductive organs, also termed the gonads or primary reproductive organs, are designed to produce, nurture, store and release mature gametes (ova and spermatozoa). They also secrete steroid hormones called sex hormones (primarily testosterone in males and estrogen/progesterone in females).

The external genitalia are designed to bring the gametes in close approximation within the female reproductive tract and achieve internal fertilization.

THE FEMALE GENITAL SYSTEM

This essentially is comprised of two ovaries (A), two fallopian tubes (B), the uterus (C), vagina (D), and the perineum on the outside called the vulva. In addition is the human breasts called mammary glands.

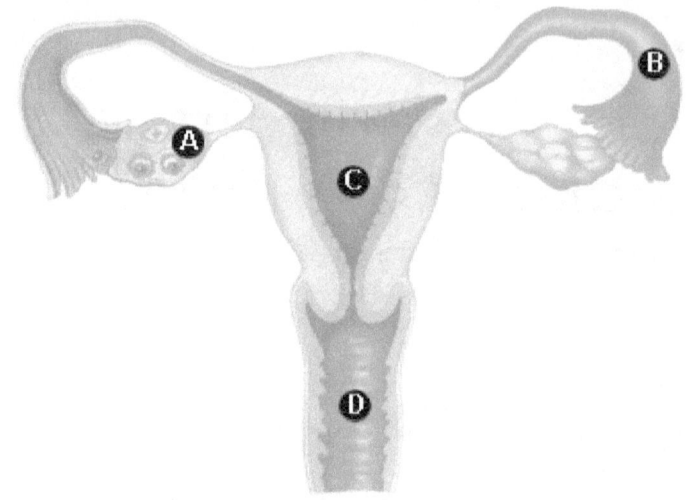

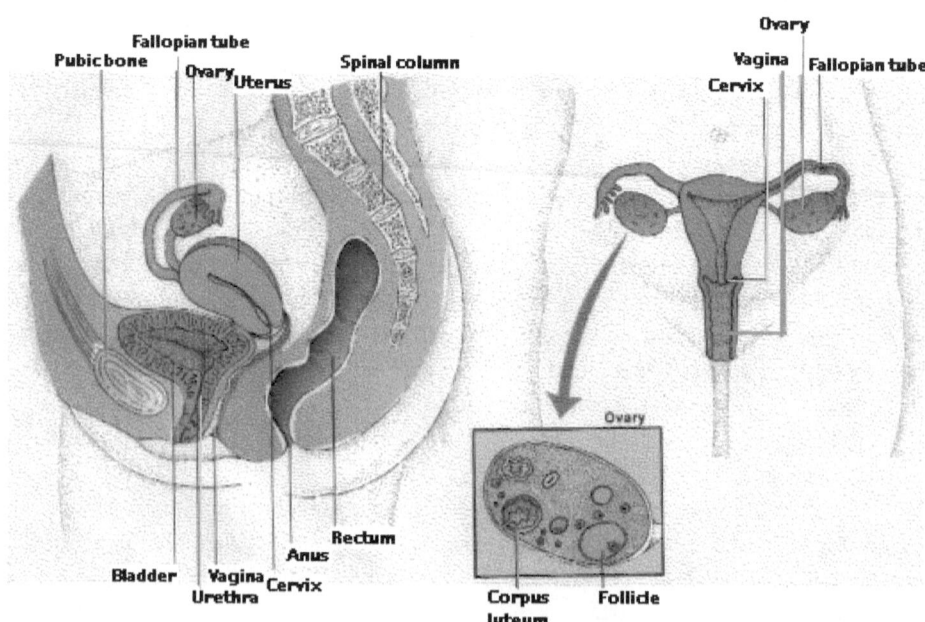

Gamete (ovum) production as well as female hormone production is the responsibility of the paired ovaries while the protection and nourishment of the developing fetus are the functions of the uterus. The breasts continue with the nourishment after the baby is born. The paired fallopian tubes provide a pathway for the eggs to transit into the uterus during fertilization and then transit of the developing embryo. The vagina is a hollow muscular tube connecting the uterus to the outside. It therefore receives semen from an erect penis during sexual intercourse as well as allows passage of menstrual flow and developed fetus from the uterus to the outside.

In sum, the female genital system is designed for the following functions:

- Produces, stores, and nurtures the eggs
- Secretes the sex hormones
- Receives the male sperms during copulation
- Protects, nourishes, and grows the fertilized egg until delivery
- Enables delivery through the birth canal
- Provides ongoing nourishment after birth via breast-feeding.

THE MALE GENITAL SYSTEM

For descriptive purposes, this can be divided into four parts labeled 1-6 below.

A. Testes (2)—the male gonads that produce spermatozoa (spermatogenesis).

B. Epididymis (3) and vas deferens (4)—organs that mature, store, and transport the spermatozoa.

C. The accessory sex glands—the prostate (6), seminal vesicles (5) supply the fluid (seminal plasma) of the semen. Prostatic secretion (about 30-35% of semen) is acidic, containing proteolytic enzymes that liquefy the ejaculate within twenty to twenty-five minutes of release while seminal vesicle fluid (about 65% of semen) is alkaline and rich in fructose and protein kinase, which coagulates the ejaculate on release.

D. Penis (1)—the male organ for copulation and delivery of semen to the female.

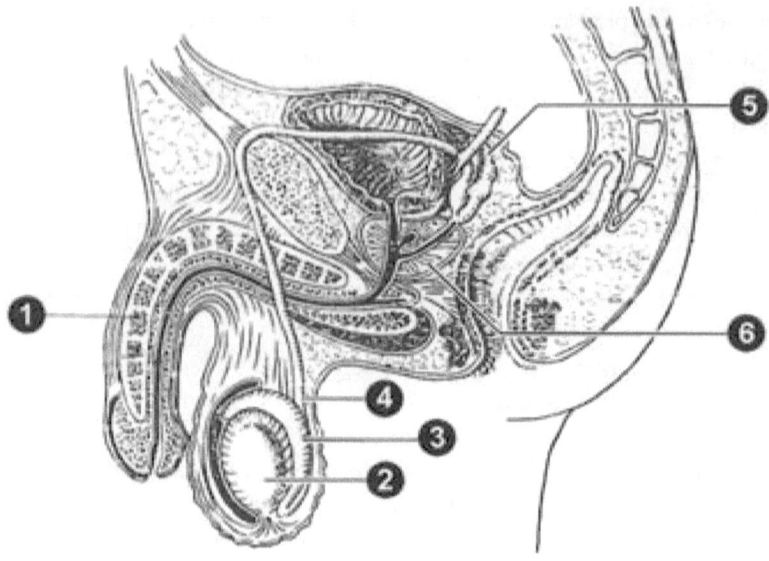

Gametogenesis

This is the process of developing the reproductive cells termed gametes (spermatozoa in males and ova in females).

The predecessor cells of the gametes termed the primordial germ cells begin their differentiation very early in intrauterine life! In fact, by the third week in utero, primordial germ cells are already differentiated from the somatic progenitor ectodermal cells and begin their migration via the extra embryonic endoderm into the site of the future gonads called the gonadal ridge. This occurs by the fifth week in utero. At the stage, the gonad is indeterminate, that is, no difference between the male and female gonad. Then the presence or absence of Y chromosomes initiates sexual differentiation of the gonads between the seventh and ninth week of intrauterine life.

Once the definite gonads are formed, there is then marked variations, especially in timings in this process of gametogenesis between human males and females.

With respect to female gametogenesis or oogenesis, this is initiated in utero. The maximum number of oogonia present in both ovaries (6 to 7 million) is established by the fifth-month gestation. These oogonia are formed by the primordial germ cells multiplying by simple mitosis. Thereafter, their number starts to deplete by atresia in a process termed apoptosis, initially very rapidly to birth when only about 2 million are present and then more slowly after birth until menopause. By puberty, the number has declined to only about three hundred thousand to four hundred thousand oocytes. Of these, only about four hundred oocytes are destined to be ovulated during the woman's reproductive lifetime; the rest also undergo atresia.

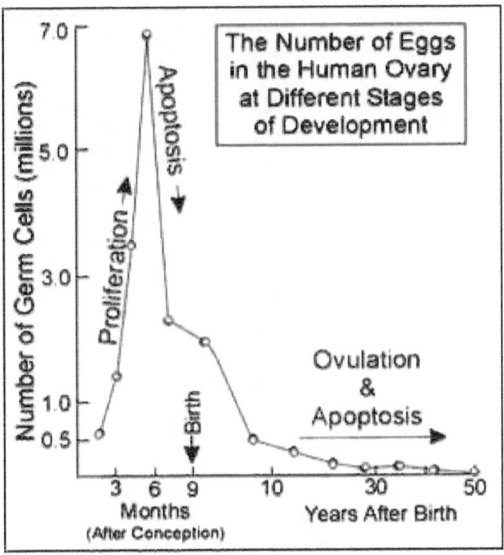

Thus, all the woman's eggs are completely formed during fetal development. In fact, it has been established that by the twelfth week of intrauterine life, the very first primary oocytes are already being formed by the oogonia entering the prophase 1 of meiosis, accompanied by the restructuring of the surrounding coelomic epithelial covering to form the primordial follicles with the primary oocytes arrested in the dictyotene stage of prophase 1 of meiosis. This transformation involving the development and maturation of the ova and their surrounding follicular cells forming the primordial follicles take approximately four weeks and is described as oogenesis and follicular development.

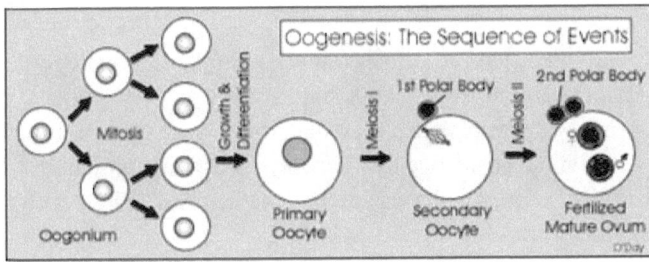

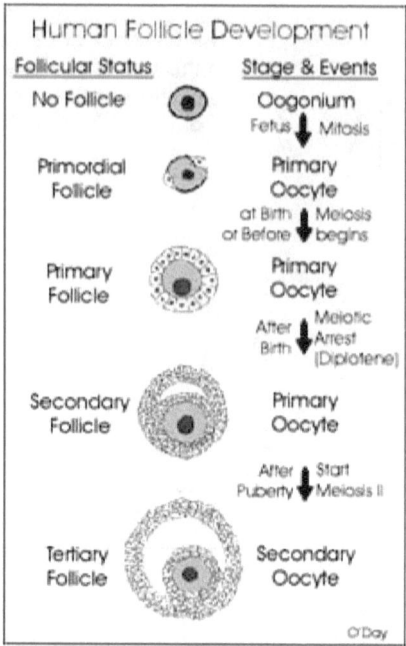

For male gametogenesis or spermatogenesis, this does not commence until puberty but, once established, appears to continue throughout the man's life. After gonadal differentiation in utero and the formation of spermatogonia by mitosis, further development begins at puberty under the influence of testosterone among other factors, leading to the formation of spermatozoa. This takes approximately sixty-four days to accomplish:

- An initial three steps of mitosis transforming the spermatogonia into primary spermatocytes. This takes about sixteen days.
- The primary spermatocytes then undergoes meiosis 1 in a rather prolonged process lasting up to twenty-four days and with prophase 1 with its five histological distinct phases lasting the longest. The result is secondary spermatocytes.
- The secondary spermatocytes are rather endangered and therefore rapidly undergo meiosis 2. The brief duration (only a few hours, about five hours) of meiosis 2 is because neither synthesis of DNA nor a new grouping of chromosomes takes place here. The results are haploid cells called spermatids.
- Finally, there is the differentiation of spermatids into spermatozoa in a complex process lasting about twenty-four days. This process is otherwise termed spermiogenesis, resulting in mature spermatozoa comprising the head, neck, and long tail.

The whole process takes place in waves and averages about 100 million sperms per day.

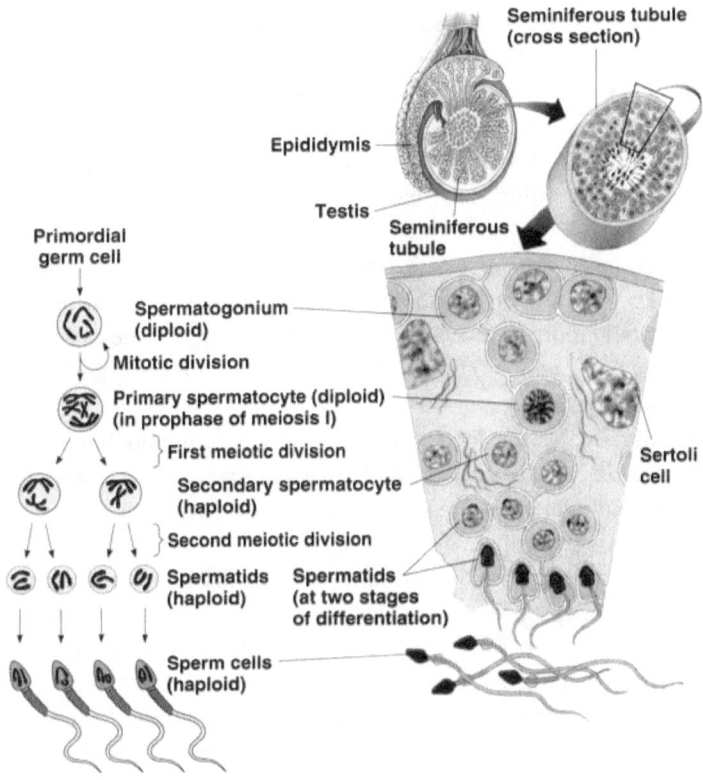

Note how the above help explain some of the differences between spermatogenesis and oogenesis, including why age appears to have a major role in females' fertility compared to the males'!

Firstly, there is no male germ cell production in utero and, as such, no meiosis in utero unlike the entire female germ cells, which are all formed from meiosis in utero.

Next in spermatogenesis, one primary spermatocyte gives rise to four spermatids with its cytoplasm equally divided between each spermatid while in oogenesis, one primary oocyte forms only one mature ovum at the end of meiosis 2, which receives all the cytoplasm of the primary oocyte (a large cell of about 120 microns) with consequent release of two small daughter cells containing only unwanted chromosomes (termed polar bodies). Thus, only about four hundred ova reach maturity and get ovulated during the entire woman's reproductive life by completing the first meiotic division, releasing the first polar body and entering the second meiotic division until metaphase when it is once again arrested. Once fertilization occurs, the second meiotic division is completed, and the second polar body is then extruded.

Ovulation

This is seen in the females involving the shedding of the ovum from the ovary, initiated at puberty. As the follicle matures, it enlarges, reaching 15-18 mm in size and, at same time, approximates to the surface of the ovary. A combination of factors such as high LH level, increased activity of collagenase enzymes and enzymatic digestion, increased PG levels, and increased follicular fluid pressure all working together lead to ovulation by such effects as the stroma and theca becoming very thin, an avascular area (stigma) appearing at the most convex point in the follicle while the cells of the cumulus oophorus becoming loosened with the accumulation of intercellular fluids between them.

Once ovulation has occurred, the fate of the ovum is decided by fertilization; otherwise, it dies within twelve to thirty hours. In vivo in humans, the fimbria of the fallopian tube would more or less embrace the ovary such that the ovum is carried into the tube partly by the accompanying discharged follicular fluid and partly by the activity of ciliated cells lining the tube.

Note specifically that the shed ovum is still not fully mature but only a secondary oocyte measuring about 100 microns and a distinct perivitalline space containing the first polar body. No nucleus is present as the nuclear membrane had been dissolved. Rather, the spindle is present.

It is also important to note the formation of a vitally important organ that rapidly develops from the collapsed follicle left behind in the ovary at ovulation termed corpus luteum (yellow body). It is formed from the follicular cells and some theca internal cells, which increase in size, acquire polyhedral shape with cytoplasm filled with yellow pigments called lutein, and begin secreting progesterone and some estrogen. Its fate is also determined by fertilization. If there is fertilization, it is called corpus luteum of pregnancy, continues to increase in size, secreting more progesterone and persisting for up to four months. If there is no fertilization, it is called corpus luteum of menstruation and lasts only two weeks before it degenerates, forming white fibrous mass termed corpus albicantes.

Cyclic changes in certain hormones of the hypothalamo-pituitary ovarian system are responsible for the periodicity of follicle maturation and ovulation in the ovaries termed the ovarian cycle as well as the concurrent cyclical alterations in the endometrial lining of the uterus termed the menstrual cycle.

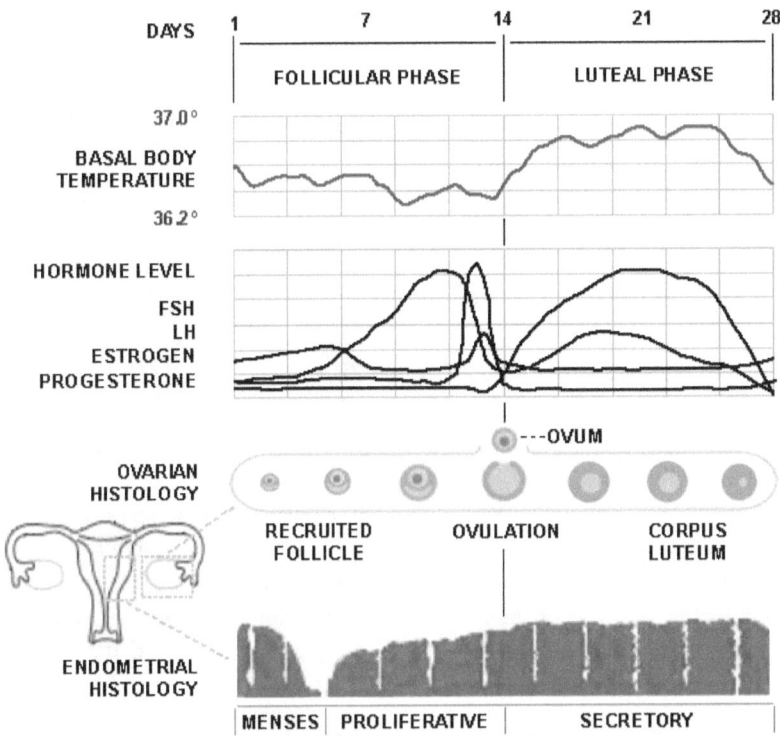

PRENATAL DEVELOPMENT

Fertilization

When viable female eggs and male sperms are brought into close proximity either during copulation or artificially within the female reproductive system as occurs during insemination or even in the test tube as occurs during IVF, the result is fertilization. This is essentially the penetration of the egg with the sperm and subsequent fusion of their genetic material to form an embryo. This involves a sequence of events, which, for descriptive purposes, could be said to involve the following steps:

1. Capacitation of the sperms, which occurs in vivo in the female genital tract, whereby the sperms undergo a series of metabolic and membrane-associated changes in order to be able to fertilize the egg.

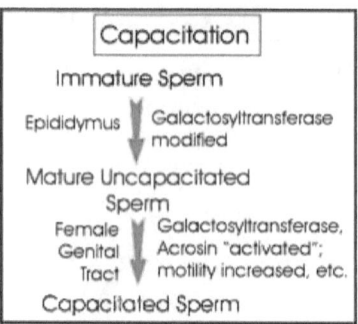

2. Binding of the sperms to ZP2 in the ZP.
3. Acrosome reaction triggered by the binding of the sperms to the ZP, which aims to mobilize enzymes with the head of the spermatozoon to degrade the zona pellucida.
4. Cortical reaction now involving the secondary oocyte, whose cortical granules release enzymes by exocytosis to the ZP, causing the glycoprotein in the ZP to cross-link with each other and thus impermeable to other sperms. This prevents fertilization of an egg by more than one sperm. Furthermore, the cortical reaction triggers second meiotic division, producing the haploid ovum and releasing the second polar body.

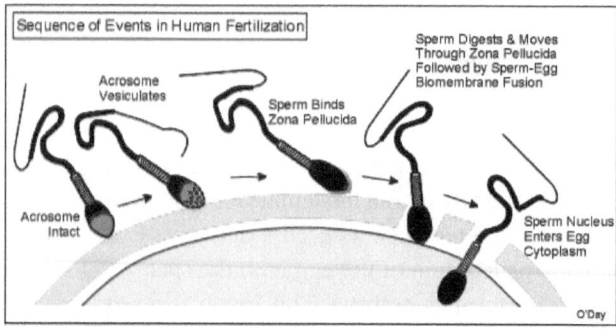

5. Fusion of the sperm with the egg, whereby the cell membranes of the secondary oocyte and sperm fuse.

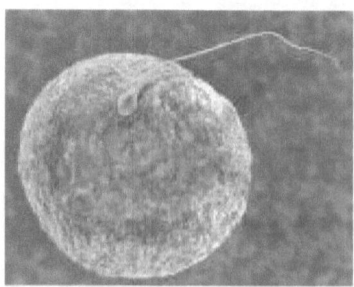

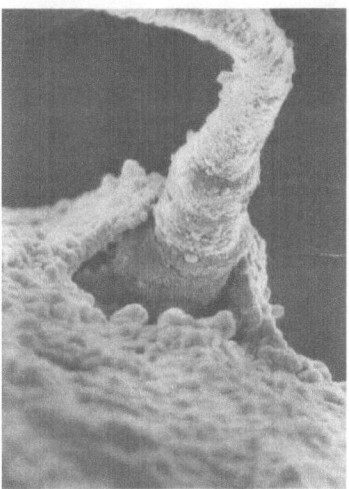

In vivo, this usually occurs in the ampullary region of the fallopian tube, and although 20-250 million sperms are normally deposited in the upper vagina, the numbers diminish rapidly during movement in the female genital tract, thus the following occurs:

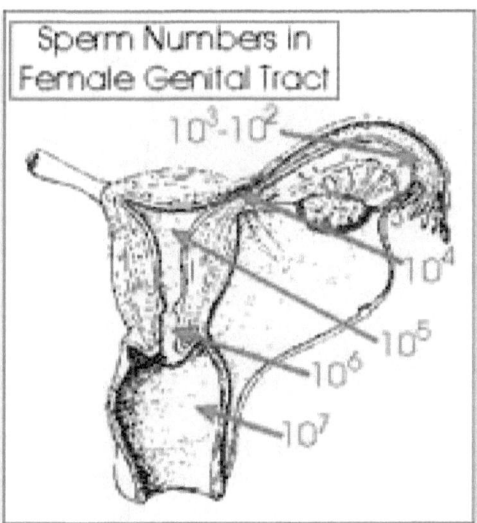

Sperm Numbers in Female Genital Tract

10^3-10^2
10^4
10^5
10^6
10^7

6. Transformation and mitosis, whereby the genetic materials of both the sperm and egg undergo transformations with the formation of the pronuclei and migration toward the center of the oocyte, the dissolution of the pronuclei membranes, and then mitosis restoring the diploid state and forming the zygote. The sperm's tail and mitochondria degenerate such that all the mitochondria of the embryo are of maternal origin.

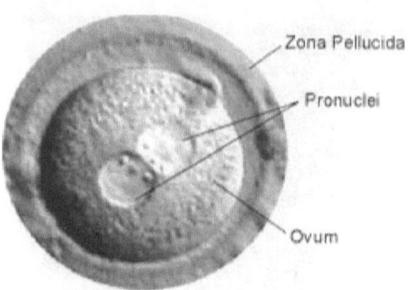

After fertilization and subsequent formation of the zygote, embryogenesis starts until the tenth week of gestation (or eighth week of intrauterine life (IUL)) when the precursors of all the major organs are laid down. This zygote begins cell division by mitosis to form the embryo, initially forming a ball of cells called morula and then fluid accumulation within the morula to form cavity and transformation into a blastocyst. Meanwhile, and up till this stage, there is no overall increase in the size of the embryo compared with the fertilized ovum as each successive cell division produces smaller cells even as the embryo is traveling down the fallopian tube toward the endometrial cavity.

By the fifth day after fertilization or third week of gestation, the embryo reaches the endometrial cavity and begins the process of implantation.

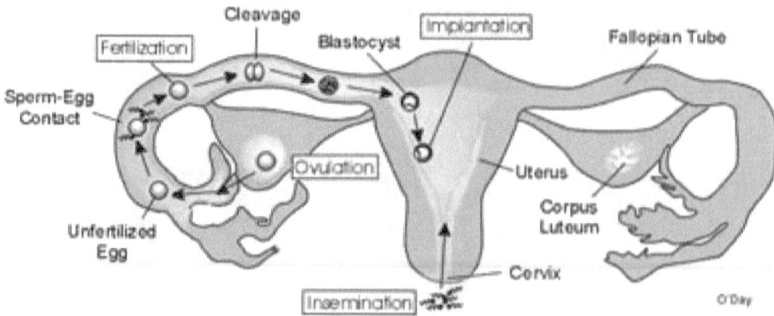

Implantation

This is arguably the most critical stage in the establishment of pregnancy, involving a complex series of synchronous events of both the conceptus and the endometrium occurring over time. It has been variously estimated that between 30 and 70% are lost before or at the time of implantation, most often without the woman even being aware that she is pregnant (Cook 1088)!

For descriptive purposes, the implantation of human embryo, which in vivo would occur at the blastocyst stage, could again be seen as involving these stages:

1. Synchronization of the embryo-endometrium development via extensive paracrine cross talk between the blastocyst and the endometrium

2. Lysis of the ZP—the glycoprotein shell—enabling contact and attachment of the trophectoderm to the luminal epithelium of the endometrium by the interaction of adhesion molecules and their receptors
3. The penetration of the epithelial cell layer of the endometrium, the basement membrane, and the invasion of the underlying stroma

Recent studies have shown that implantation is likely mediated via a number of signaling and adhesion molecules, although the precise molecular mechanisms involved in the humans are not understood (Bischof P et al, 2000). Presently, most of our knowledge about the physiology of implantation is from animal experiments as ethical reasons preludes most studies in humans, but it is still being hoped that IVF-ET would throw some more light even as the low embryo implantation with these advanced technologies has remained a major concern.

In most successful pregnancies, the embryo implants by eight to ten days after ovulation (Wilcox AJ et al, 1999).

Differentiation
With successful implantation, rapid growth occurs with the production of the different cell types in a process called differentiation. The initial part of this process is termed gastrulation, resulting in the establishment of the three germ layers—the ectoderm, mesoderm, and endoderm, followed by embryogenesis when the various organ systems are differentiated. This is completed by the tenth week of gestation or eighth week of IUL.

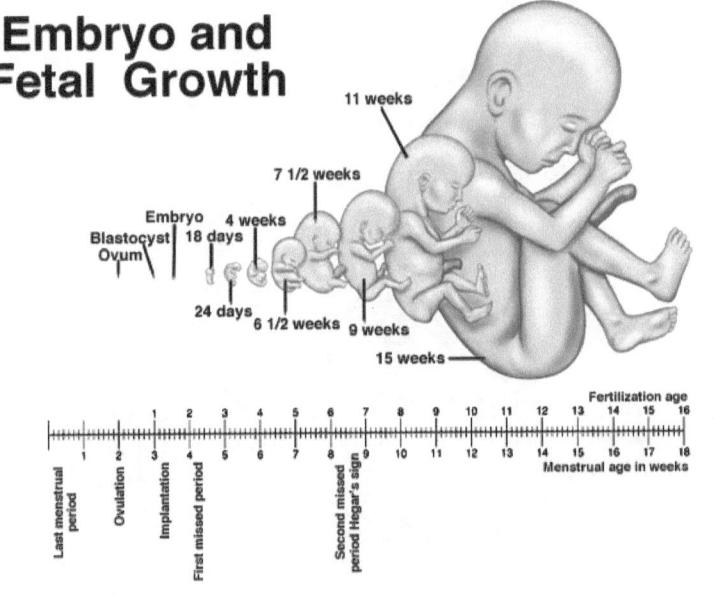

Thereafter, the remainder of human development in utero is termed fetal development, characterized by continuing rapid growth and tissue differentiation. It is during this phase that the human fetus becomes recognizable as human.

Parturition

This is the final step in pregnancy, otherwise called labor or childbirth and is traditionally divided into three stages:

First stage: shortening and dilatation of cervix

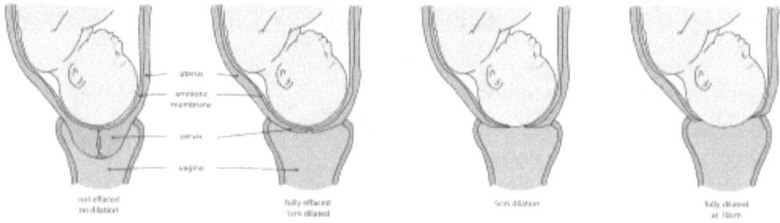

Second stage: descent and delivery of the newborn

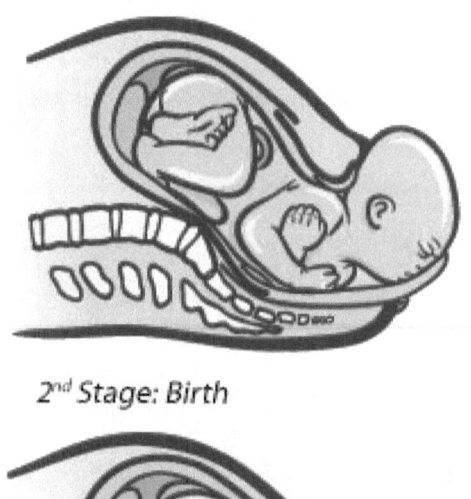

2ⁿᵈ Stage: Birth

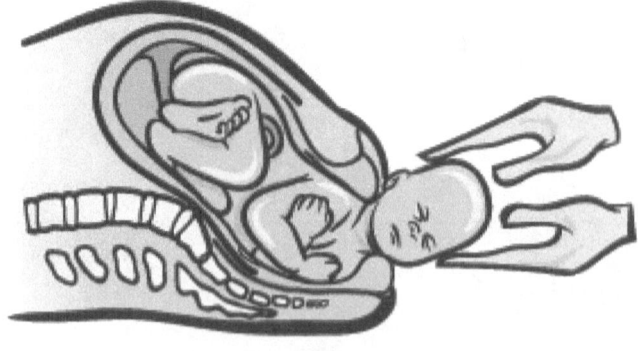

Third stage: delivery of the placenta

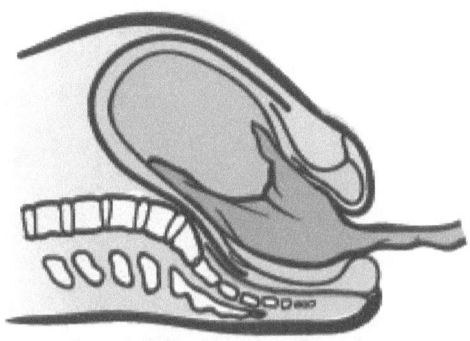

3ʳᵈ Stage Placenta Expulsion

Since the nineteenth century, the following stages can be interrupted at any stage by operative delivery termed cesarean section while the second stage by instrumental delivery (forceps or vacuum delivery).

The exact mechanism initiating human parturition has remained elusive with different theories suggesting either the placenta or the fetus or the mother or a combination of either of them which then initiates a cascade of biochemical reaction that ultimately results in labor. Further details are beyond the scope of this book. However, it is important to note that but for successful, timely initiation and conduct of parturition that is tightly regulated, both premature and postmature deliveries could result in increased perinatal mortality and morbidity.

POSTNATAL DEVELOPMENT

Postdelivery, the newborn immediately enters the neonatal period—the first twenty-eight days of life. The immediate challenge at birth is the successful conversion of fetal cardiopulmonary status to the norm postdelivery. This involves tremendous respiratory and hemodynamic changes beyond the scope of this book. There are some immediate adaptation changes in the mother. The next challenge is feeding and bonding of the newborn with the mother. There is also the continuing growth and development of all organ systems of the body, especially the brain and central nervous system.

Other periods thereafter include infancy (one month to two years of life), childhood (two years to adolescence), adolescence (age twelve or thirteen to adulthood or maturity), and finally, maturity thereafter until old age and death. The process of aging is called senescence.

Chapter 3

ASSESSMENT OF THE INFERTILE COUPLE

My life seems on hold . . . except for continuing medical tests,
appointments, and treatments . . . I hate not having definite
answers or guarantees.

—the infertile

An optimal assessment of the infertile couple should be timely, reliable, accurate, cost-effective, and possibly minimally invasive as well as providing the physician with useful prognostic information for all possible treatment options.

Therefore, the first priority is timely intervention as it has been well established that maternal age is a major determinant for pregnancy rates. Furthermore, by the time individuals/couples present themselves for treatment, they are usually very anxious to get started on their evaluations and treatment promptly!

Detailed and focused history/examination/investigations should ideally be obtained from the couple, thus the following:

Female	Male
History	
Duration of infertility	Same
Fertility/prior pregnancies in other relationships	Same
Gynecologic Hx	Hx of coital habits

Menstrual history: age at menarche, cycle length and regularity, and other symptoms suggestive of ovulation like mittelschmerz pains, dysmenorrhea

Erectile dysfunction, spontaneous erections/ejaculations and dysfunctions

Hx of PID, fibroids, cervical dysplasias, IUCD use

Same as applicable

Sexual dysfunction, frequency of intercourse

Previous surgical Hx, including hydroceles, varicoceles, inguinal

Previous pelvic-abdominal surgeries

hernias, torsion, cryptorchidism, etc.

Medications, including prior contraception use

Same

Smoking/drugs/alcohol use

Same

Environmental exposures, including DES, radiations, etc.

Excessive heat, chemical, radiations, etc.

Physical examinations with special emphasis on the following

Weight, height, BMI, BP, pallor

same

Breast examination, including stage, nipples, size, galactorrhea, and other secondary sexual characteristics like build, hair distribution, etc.

Same

Abdominal examination

Same

Genitourinary system/pelvic examination, especially external genitalia and pelvic organs

Genitourinary system/rectal examination, especially testicular size and tumors/ cysts and prostate examination

The volume of the testicle (normal 15-35 ml)

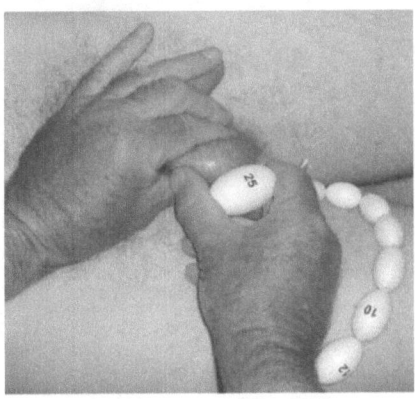

Other systems including CNS examination, including visual field defect respiratory system

Same + anosmia (Kallmann's syndrome) chronic sinusitis and bronchiectasis (Young's syndrome, Kartagener's syndrome)

Baseline Investigations

Day 3 hormonal profile, including serum FSH, LH, E2, prolactin, testosterone, and TSH
midluteal phase progesterone

Baseline FSH, LH, prolactin, and TSH

Semen analysis (SA)*
This is the basic test in the male fertility workup even prior to any blood hormonal tests. It provides important clinical information on spermatogenesis, function competence of spermatozoa as well as the secretionary pattern of male accessory glands. (See below for details, current WHO guidelines.*) All these aid in the determination of the spermatozoon fertility potential.

Pelvic US

Testicular/scrotal US

Used mostly in imaging internal female pelvic structures, especially the ovaries, uterus, and even the tubes in cases of hydrosalpinges

Especially for testicular volume and other anomalies including orchitis, epididymo-orchitis, varicocele, spermatocele, epididyal cysts, and undescended testes

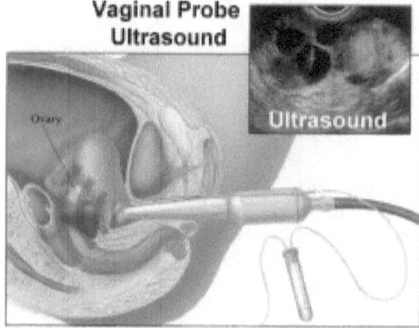

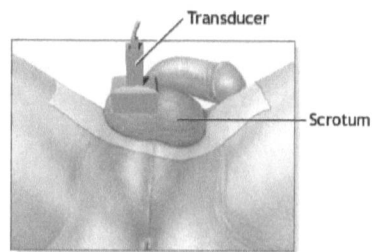

Tubal Patency Test (e.g., Sono HSG, HSG)

This uses either x-rays or US to study the uterine cavity as well as give a basic assessment of tubal patency.

*SA (WHO 2010) Criteria

Minimum requirements for SA and its parameters had long been a subject of great debate, necessitating WHO's attempts to standardize SA protocols and standards with its publication manuals initially in 1980, then 1987, 1992, 1999, and the latest, the fifth edition, in 2010, thus:

volume	=	>=2mls
pH	=	<7.2
concentration	=	>=15x10`6/ml
total count	=	>=40million/ejaculate
motility	=	>=40% total motility
And	>=	32% progressive motility within sixty minutes of ejaculation
morphology	=	>=4% with normal morphology and form
WBC	=	<1x10`6/ml
immunobead test	=	<50% spermatozoa with adherent particles
MAR test	=	<50% spermatozoa with adherent particles

The following are special conditions to be met:
1. Two to seven days' abstinence from sexual intercourse.
2. Semen should be obtained by masturbation into a sterile wide-mouth container.
3. SA should be performed within one hour of semen collection.

SA-MACROSCOPY

A normal semen has a gray-opalescent appearance. The ejaculate is initially coagulated and, within the hour, liquefies.

The total volume should be 2 ml or more (usually between 2 and 7 ml) with sperms constituting about 10% of this volume.

The pH should be more than 7.2. A lower pH is often seen with low sperm counts or malformation of the male reproductive tract.

SA-MICROSCOPY

Sperm count could be done either manually or by computer (CASA), providing both the concentration and the total count.

Both sperm motility and morphology provide the best criteria for demonstrating the fertilizing capacity of the sperms; the sperm motility gives a measure of the integrity of the sperm axoneme and tail structure as well as the metabolic machinery of the mitochondria while the morphology gives a measure of the integrity of DNA packaging as well as the quality of spermatogenesis. Between these two parameters, the jury is still out although the consensus is that morphology is probably the most important SA parameter with respect to natural fertilization (Bartoov B et al, 1994), IUI (Berkovitz A et al, 1999), and routine IVF (Kruger TF et al, 1988; Mashiach R et al, 1992).

High leukocytes indicate infection-necessitating cultures for aerobic and anaerobic organisms well as for chlamydia and mycoplasma. Additionally, WBCs also have the ability to release ROS (superoxide anions, hydrogen peroxides, and hydroxyl radicals), which inhibit sperm motility and sperm function.

If a semen sample falls within the WHO range, the ejaculate is described as normozoospermia. Otherwise, various terminologies are applicable to different anomalies such as the following:

oligozoospermia = sperm concentration of less than 15 million sperms per milliliter

azoospermia = no spermatozoa in the ejaculate or retrograde ejaculation

aspermia = no ejaculate or no sperm volume

hypospermia = semen volume < 2.0mls

hyperspermia = semen volume > 7.0mls

asthenozoospermia = sperm motility <50%

teratozospermia = <14% normal forms

necrozoospermia = only nonviable (dead) sperms

pyospermia = leukocytes >1x10'6 WBCs/ml

hematospermia = presence of RBCs in semen

oligoasthenoteratozoospermia syndrome (OATS) = where the three pathologies occur simultaneously as often is the case!

OTHER INVESTIGATIONS

Other relevant tests based on findings from history and physical examination—such as diabetes screen; autoimmune diseases, including antiphospholipid antibody syndrome; various endocrine disorders, etc.—could also be initiated as well as some specialized investigations such as the following:

Diagnostic Laparoscopy

This is an invasive procedure performed under a general anesthesia mainly to further diagnose tubal and other intrapelvic causes of infertility for which it is still the gold standard. However, most modern infertility management precludes its routine use because of its invasiveness, using instead HSG/Sono HSG to confirm tubal patency; otherwise, either IVF and/or ICSI could be planned thereafter if tubal occlusion is confirmed. It has, however, remained the gold standard in the diagnosis and management of endometriosis.

Laparoscopic Procedure

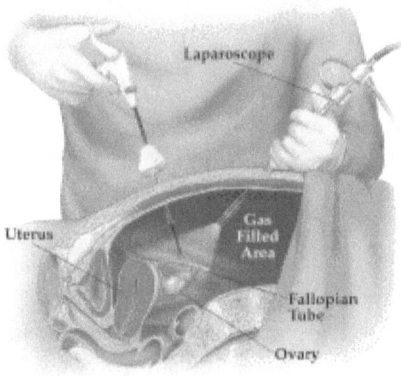

Endometrial Biopsy

This is an office procedure used to obtain endometrial lining for histological examination. When timed appropriately, it could document ovulation as well as assess the endometrial status with respect to implantation. Thus, it could aid the diagnosis of LPD. Its routine use in clinical practice is still controversial and probably not cost-effective (Coutifaris C et al, 2004).

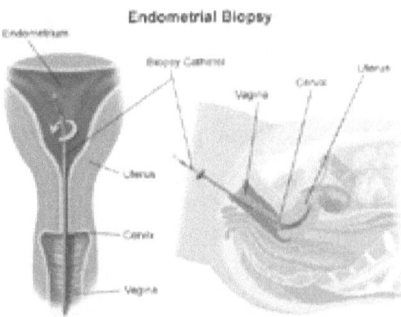

Tests of Ovarian Reserve

Screening for ovarian reserve is a fundamental component of female infertility investigations as they attempt to describe the native oocyte endowment and thus is closely related to the woman's reproductive potential. Accurate and reliable assessment of ovarian reserve also predicts successful ovarian stimulation during ART and possible stimulation protocol modifications to enhance success (Jayaprakasan BK et al, 2008). Several tests for ovarian reserve have been developed in clinical practice over the past few decades for ovarian reserve, either directly on the ovaries by assessment using ultrasound (antral follicular sound (Tomas C et al, 1997) and ovarian volume (Lass A et al, 1997)) or indirectly by measurement of serum hormones produced by the follicles estradiol (Smotrich DB et al, 1995), inhibin B (Seifer DB et al, 1999), anti-Müllerian hormone (van Rooij JA et al, 1999) and the hormones under inhibitory control of the hormones FSH (sharif K et al, 1998), LH (Weghofer A et al, 2006), namely day 3 FSH or basal FSH level.

Already mentioned above as one of the routine tests, this test is actually the most commonly employed test of ovarian reserve in clinical practice. However, there remain the ongoing difficulties in establishing the absolute FSH break points compatible with achieving pregnancy (Barnhart K et al, 1999).

Hence, many other tests have been described to date to try and refine a better estimate of ovarian reserve, including the following:

- Clomiphene citrate challenge test (CCCT)

    This is akin to a stress test on the ovaries, whereby a basal day 3 FSH is initially obtained and then 100 mg of clomiphene citrate (Clomid) is administered from days 5 to 9. Repeat serum FSH level is then obtained. A sum of the two FSH levels exceeding 25 suggests poor ovarian reserve. It is probably the best screening test for ovarian reserve.

- Day 3 estradiol (E2) level

    A number of studies have shown that high day 3 E2 levels (>60-80 pg/ml) indicate poor stimulation with few oocyte retrieval (Evers JL et al, 1998).

- Serum inhibin B level

    Low inhibin B levels (produced by "good" ovarian follicles) suggest poor ovarian response. Its clinical application is still somewhat limited because of lack of a satisfactory assay technique (Creus M et al, 2000).

- Serum anti-Müllerian hormone level (AMH)

    A glycoprotein hormone solely expressed in the females by the ovary thought to effect the transition from resting primordial into growing follicles(te Velde ER et al, 2002) and therefore could be used as a marker for ovarian reserve(de Vet et al, 2002) especially since it is noted to decline with increasing female age (Seifer DB et al, 2002)

- Antral follicular count on US

    This has been shown to provide a marker for the ovarian age that is distinct from chronological age or hormonal markers especially useful in predicting outcome in IVF procedures (Nahum R et al, 2001).

- Ovarian volume assessment

    This is usually assessed using ultrasound measurements of ovarian width, length and depth. Low ovarian volume has been found to correlate with reproductive success and higher cancellation rates in IVF cycles although widespread clinical application is still under study.

TESTS ON CERVICAL MUCUS

The Postcoital Test (PCT)

This is probably the oldest test in infertility management and involves the timed examination of a sample of cervical mucus under the microscope, collected six to twenty-four hours after intercourse. Timing is of the essence as it has to be done during the preovulatory period. A positive test in which many normal sperms are seen swimming in the cervical mucus is very reassuring about most aspects of infertility; that is, the act of coitus is satisfactory with adequate sperms deposited in the vagina. The cervical glands are healthy and well estrogenized, suggestive of ovulation, and there are no antibodies in the mucus hostile to the sperms. Thus, a negative test has meaning only if it is repeatedly negative under a well-timed condition.

A modified PCT, sometimes termed the strict criteria in sperm morphology, is specially adapted in IVF programs based on the morphology of postcoital spermatozoa found at the level of the internal cervical os. Here, normal forms should be more than 14%. Men with fewer than 4% normal forms usually fail to fertilize without micromanipulation.

In summary, note that all the infertile couples want are babies, not just exhaustive and prolonged investigation; that is, they don't just want to know what is wrong with them but, more importantly, what can be done for them. Thus, and in consonant with the theme of this book, an optimal approach to their management commences with a pragmatic evaluation, which should be the most cost-effective protocol, especially for people in the poor countries. The baseline investigations could simply be the following:

For the woman
    day 3 FSH/LH/prolactin/TSH/estradiol
    rubella/blood group
    baseline US with sono HSG

For the man, only SA could be sufficient.

And if possible (although rare), the above management protocol should all be performed with the first consultation visit so that by the second visit, prompt treatment could be initiated unless further investigations are desired.

These are clearly illustrated in figure 1 in the next chapter.

Chapter 4

CURRENT INFERTILITY MANAGEMENT

Eventually, I am labelled "infertile" . . . It's like being sentenced for a crime you have not committed! You are sort of on a knife's edge! Even after you commence treatment, you are on a roller-coaster ride emotionally, capable of going from the very heights to the bottom with just one phone call . . . It is a psychological minefield!

—the infertile

Modern infertility treatment . . . a "miraculous" technology . . . designed as an "obstacle course!"

—Franklin S., 1997

Following a pragmatic evaluation of the infertile couple as detailed in chapter 3, it would dawn on the "apparently" healthy couple that they now have a medical diagnostic label thrust upon them. But the bottom line for the individual couple is the optimal therapeutic intervention designed to either correct or overcome both the identifiable and unidentifiable (unexplained) cause/s.

A. PREPREGNANCY MANAGEMENT

Note, however, that modern infertility management is unique among all modern medical interventions in that it provides a rare window of opportunity in the whole of clinical medicine for extensive prepregnancy counseling with maximum health education and promotion before the couple actually benefits from the results of their medical intervention, that is, before pregnancy is achieved! Thus, management of the infertile provides the clinician with an unparalleled opportunity, which ought to be mandatory, to counsel and educate the couple on the basic physiology of reproduction as well as such lifestyle changes such as smoking cessation, alcohol and caffeine reduction, etc.—all that will help to improve fertility.

Also, ancillary infertility treatments detailed below are also initiated on consultation by the infertile.

Figure 1 below is a summary of management algorithm for a cost-effective, modern, and up-to-date management of the infertile couple.

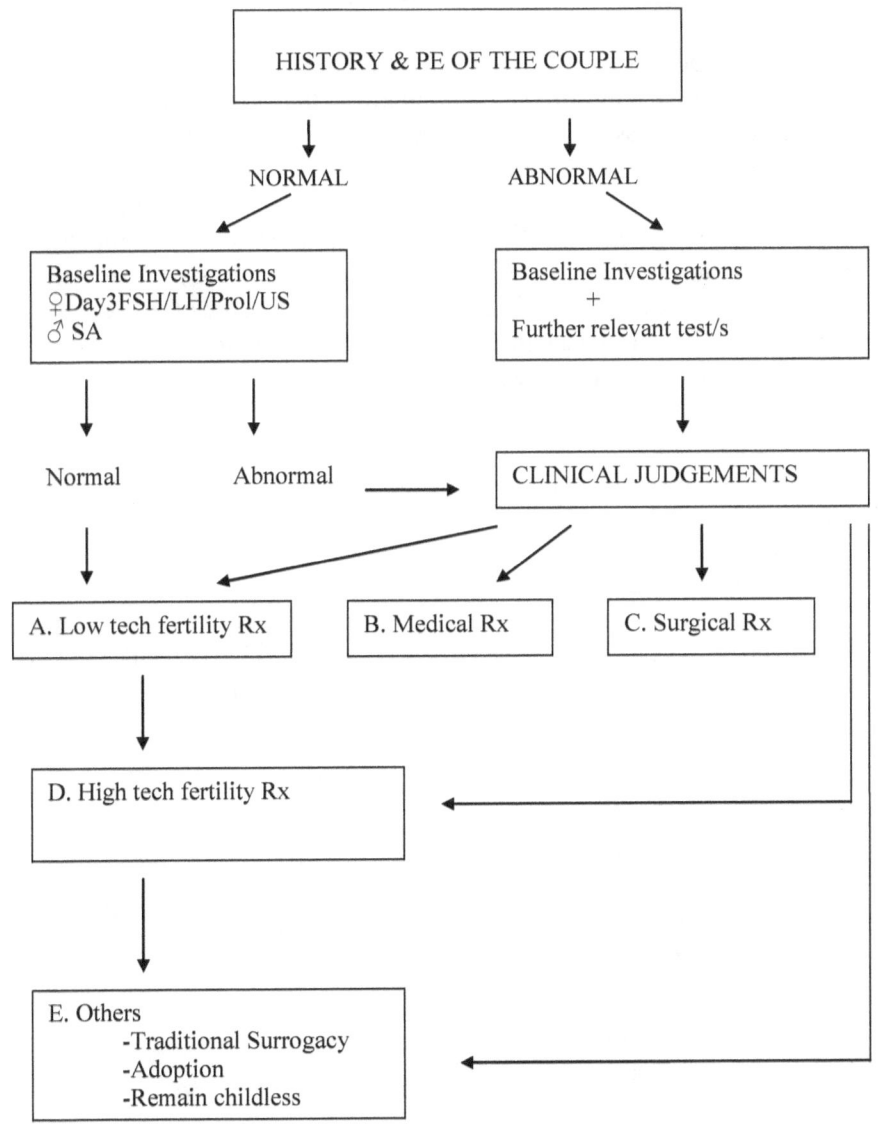

From the above, when initial evaluation (Hx, PE, and baseline investigations) are normal, a diagnosis of unexplained infertility is entertained. This diagnosis, oftentimes, can be very frustrating for the couple who may interpret this to mean that since there is no apparent cause, there is also no effective treatment! This is definitely not the case. Compatible published data have indicated that with optimal clinical judgement in the management of these cases, including where abnormalities are detected, approximately 80% of infertile couples undergoing such a treatment algorithm as above can expect to conceive (Gleicher N, 2000).

B. Low-Tech Fertility Treatments (Low-Tech ART)

TIMED INTERCOURSE

This is probably the most basic of all infertility treatment. In its simplest form, it could be applied in cases of unexplained infertility. Education, information, and counseling should be provided to all with respect to identifying ovulation, optimal timing of intercourse in relation to ovulation, and reasonable time frames for couples to achieve pregnancy given. The likeliest time to achieve pregnancy is from two days before ovulation to the day of ovulation (Wilcox AJ et al, 1995). Otherwise, some modifications could be devised ranging from rhythm method, use of cervical mucus or urine ovulation kit to time the intercourse to even more complicated cycle monitoring with ultrasound and/or HCG trigger for ovulation.

ARTIFICIAL INSEMINATIONS

This involves the artificial placement of sperms inside the woman's genital tract other than via sexual intercourse.

i.   Intrauterine insemination (IUI)
     This is currently the most widely practiced form of artificial insemination involving the placing of prepared or washed sperms (0.1-1.0 ml) in the uterine cavity with the aid of a small catheter through the cervix.

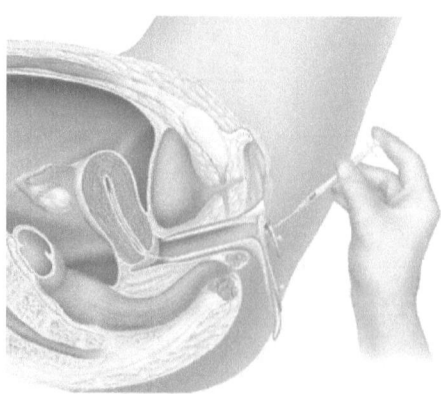

IUI was first applied in clinical practice (Lalich RA et al, 1986) as treatment for poor postcoital tests and immunologic infertility. It is a low-tech fertility treatment that theoretically allows for a relatively higher concentration of spermatozoa to reach the oocyte. The first key consideration in this fertility treatment is the type of sperm preparation method to be used, either the conventional sperm wash method or the swim up or the density gradient centrifugation method. For this, there are as yet insufficient data to recommend one method over the other for IUI (Boomsma CM et al, 2007). The next important consideration is timing of the IUI. Here, there is ample evidence that the use of cheaper urinary LH detection rather than HCG injection is more practical and more cost-effective when clomiphene citrate is used for ovarian stimulation (Kosmas IP et al, 2007). The final consideration is the number of inseminations per cycle. To date, most available evidence failed to show increased efficacy with double IUI compared with single IUI per ovulatory cycle (NICE guidelines 2004; Osuna C et al, 2004).

In recent times, the indications for IUI have been expanded to include such male and female disorders as severe hypospadias; retrograde ejaculation; impotence; vaginismus; some mild, moderate, and even severe male factor infertility with donor sperms' IUI; as well as a routine first-line Rx for unexplained infertility.

Various variations in treatment protocols could be applied with modern IUI—including adjuvant ovulation induction and ovarian hyperstimulation, follicular tracking with serial ultrasound, and/or HCG injection to induce ovulation, donor sperm IUI, etc.—all which appear to enhance its efficacy. A large randomized study in the USA confirmed the effectiveness of IUI combined with ovarian hyperstimulation (Guzick DS et al, 1999), and this is now currently very widely practiced in most fertility clinics.

There is a lot of evidence to suggest that oral clomiphene therapy combined with IUI or natural-cycle IUI is satisfactory first-line choices of treatment for unexplained infertility and male factor infertility in low-tech settings (Abdelkader AM et al, 2009) most often found in resource-poor countries.

ii. Intravaginal insemination (IVI)

This is the simplest form of AI although rarely performed as it is only indicated in those rare instances where the woman's partner is unable to ejaculate within the vagina but can ejaculate by other means such as masturbation or with the aid of a penile vibrator. Both the couple should otherwise reveal no other cause for their infertility. In recent times, especially in the developed countries, lesbians are now using these but with donor sperms. In its simplest application, self-insemination is easily performed whereby the couple, in the privacy of their own home, have the male partner deliver the semen into a sterile container, which is then withdrawn into a syringe and placed high up in the vagina. The cost is only that of a sterile pot and syringe.

iii. Intracervical insemination (ICI)

Here, the sperm sample is injected directly unto the woman's cervix. Indications are essentially the same as for intravaginal insemination. However, this is usually performed by the physician or fertility specialist. Costwise, it is cheaper than IUI but more expensive than IVI.

iv. Intrauterine tuboperitoneal insemination (IUTPI)

Here, a much larger volume of prepared sperm (about 10 ml) is inseminated into the uterine cavity, the cervix being secured with a double nut bivalve speculum whose specially designed tip fits unto the cervix and prevents any leakage. The large-volume semen then advances through the rest of female genital, namely, uterine-tract cavity, fallopian tube, and POD.

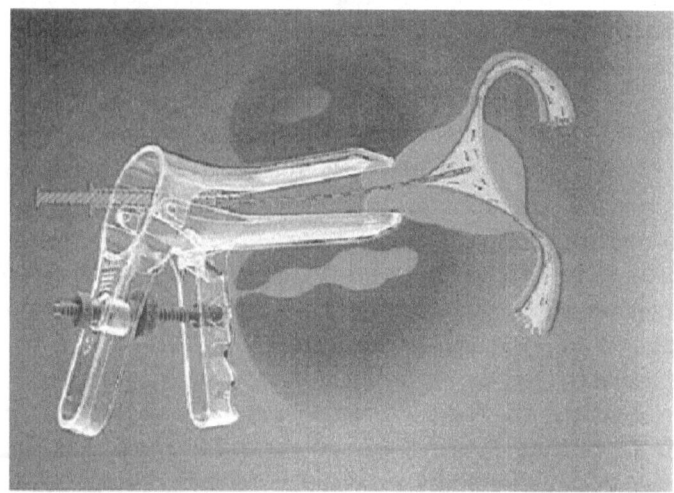

v. Intratubal insemination (ITI)

This is the most invasive form of AI and therefore most costly. It is also very rarely used, whereby sperms are deposited directly inside the fallopian tubes. There are two variants of this:

a. Intrafallopian insemination (IFI), where the prepared sperm is manipulated with the aid of a special catheter via the vagina, cervix, uterine cavity, and then into one or both tubes.

b. Sperm intrafallopian transfer (SIFT), a more invasive and time-consuming technique utilizing general anesthesia and laparoscopic surgery just like in GIFT.

Recent studies have not revealed superior benefits than IUI, especially when the additional costs are taken into consideration. Ectopic pregnancy risks are also a major consideration.

vi. Donor sperm insemination (DI)

This is essentially an IUI procedure but with donor sperms. It is therefore usually indicated when there are azoospermia or severe oligozoospermia that pregnancy is unlikely. Such conditions could result from testicular trauma, genetic defects, or iatrogenic causes such as orchidectomy or cancer therapies with radiation. Also, single women or lesbians seeking a pregnancy could use this method.

Donors can be known (designated donor) or anonymous (commercial donor programs).

Ideally, rigorous screening for medical and genetic diseases is mandatory for all donors such that frozen donor sperm should be the norm. Designated donor programs appear to be more utilized in resource-poor developing countries while commercial donor sperm services is more readily available and utilized in most developed countries.

Note well that this therapeutic DI is by far the most successful and cost-effective form of therapy for couples with male factor infertility!

Gamete Intrafallopian Transfer (GIFT)

This is a form of low-tech fertility treatment, albeit expensive, involving the initial first four steps of standard IVF-ET protocol. (See detailed outline below.)

The difference commences at step 5, where instead of insemination in a dish in a laboratory, the eggs (usually two) and sperms are placed in a catheter and injected into the fallopian tube during a laparoscopic procedure. Thus, fertilization and early embryo are hoped to occur in the natural environment of the tube and womb rather than the more high-tech laboratory of dishes and culture media. It is of note that this is one of the fertility treatment procedures officially recognized by the Roman Catholic Church. The main disadvantages include the need for patent tubes (and therefore not applicable to the many cases of blocked fallopian tubes in the third world countries), failure to confirm fertilization in a dish, and high costs, including need for GA and laparoscopy.

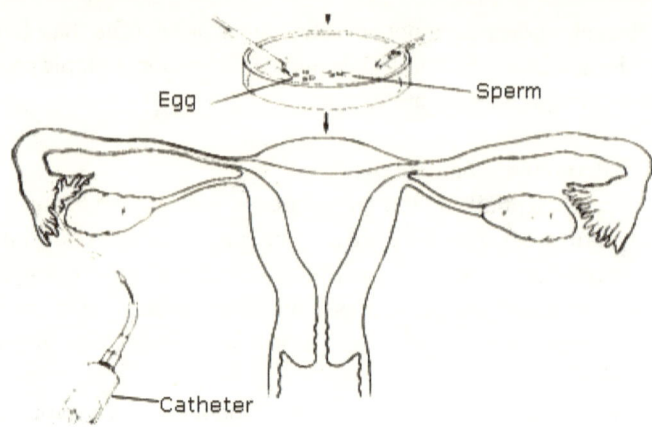

Traditional Surrogacy

The term *surrogacy* implies substitute, that is, substitute mother.

There are two main types: traditional surrogacy and gestational surrogacy.

Traditional surrogacy or the straight method is a low-tech fertility solution where the woman is pregnant with her own child but with the notion to relinquish the child to be raised by others. In fact, the story in Genesis where Rachel asked her maid to conceive a child for her by Jacob was probably the first recorded story of traditional surrogacy. The Jewish custom at the time of Jesus Christ insists on the widow being remarried to the late husband's closest male relative. (Recall the question put to Christ about a man who married a woman and dies, and the woman in turn got married to the other remaining seven brothers!) In Igbo community of Nigeria, this has also been in practice, whereby if a man dies without a child or a male heir, the wife could continue to bear children for the late husband, preferably from the late husband's close male relatives like brothers, etc. In some cases, the daughters are contracted to provide children, be it male heirs for the late fathers. Thus, this form of surrogacy appears indigenous to many cultures. In modern times, the child could be conceived either by natural sexual intercourse or by medical intervention such as IUI or other ART procedures.

Gestational surrogacy is usually carried out in conjunction with ART and therefore is treated more fully as a high-tech fertility treatment below.

C. MEDICAL TREATMENTS

FOR FEMALE FACTORS

1. Treatment for ovulatory dysfunction

The most common medically treated cause of female infertility is ovulatory dysfunction. These are often associated with a favorable outcome and includes such treatments as the following:

i.   Medications used to stimulate ovulation
-    Clomiphene citrate (CC, Serophene, Clomid, etc): A selective estrogen receptor modulator (SERM) like tamoxifen, which interferes with estrogen receptors. It is typically called the "fertility pill" and is usually given orally in a dose range of 50-150 mg from days 3 to 9 of the cycle. It acts centrally to increase gonadotropin secretion from the hypothalamus by inhibiting the negative feedback of estrogen. Unfortunately, peripherally on the uterus, it has some estrogenic effects such that sometimes attempts are made to counteract some of these adverse effects on cervical mucus and endometrium with the use of IUI and estrogen add-back. Other side effects include multiple pregnancies (5-10%) and OHSS (1%).

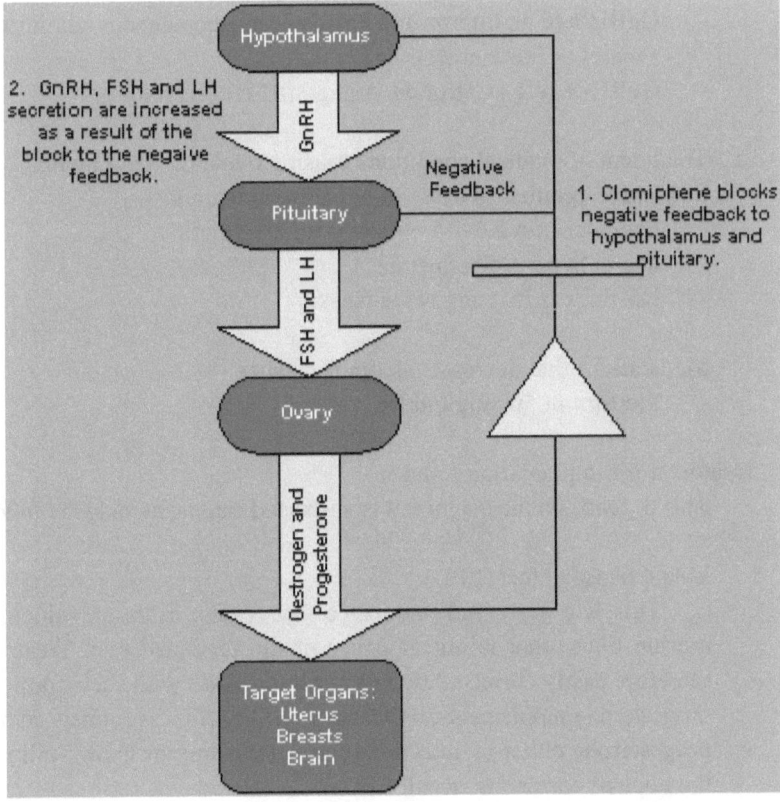

-    Letrozole (Femara): A nonsteroidal aromatase inhibitor (like anastrozole) given orally in the dose range of 2.5-5.0 mg, also from days 3 to 9. It prevents aromatase from producing estrogens by competitive reversible binding to the heme of its cytochrome P450 unit. However, and unlike CC, this group of drugs do not appear to

have an antiestrogenic effect on the endometrium and cervix such that their use may in time supersede that of the CC group.
- Gonadotrophin (Gn) therapy
E.g., HMG (e.g., personal or purified FSH (e.g., Metrodin, Follistim or Gonal-f))
These are only available as injections with exaggerated multiple pregnancy risks (25%) and OHSS (10-20%). They are generally more commonly used during ovarian hyperstimulation protocol when large quantities may be required.

ii. Medications used primarily to prevent premature ovulation
These are mostly used in conjunction with ART protocols and are mostly all available to be administered parenterally:
- GnRH-a (e.g., Lupron and Zoladex for subcutaneous administration, synarel as intranasal spray)
- GnRH-A (e.g., Cetrotide, Antagon)

iii. Treatment of medical conditions causing ovulatory dysfunction
Dopamine agonists in cases of hyperprolactinemia
- Bromocriptin 2.5-7.5 mg daily for anovulation
due to hyperprolactinemia
- Dostinex 0.25-1 mg twice weekly

Medications that decrease insulin resistance
- Metformin 500 mg bid/tid

2. Treatment for implantation failure
This depends on the diagnosed or suspected causes, namely the following:

i. Luteal phase defect (LPD)
This is a hormonal imbalance that results in the development of uterine lining that is out of phase of the fertilized egg. Treatment is therefore easily corrected by hormonal therapies with such hormones as progesterone supplements, HCG. Most fertility clinics routinely administer progesterone either by injection or as suppository or in oral-pill form in the hope of correcting occult LPD.

ii. Autoimmune/immunologic factors
Here, oral steroids are oftentimes the first-line treatment. In fact, some fertility clinics routinely administer oral steroids to all patients following ET.

iii. Treatment for recurrent miscarriage

Commonest cause is genetic/chromosomal anomalies either in terms of structure (structural anomalies) or in terms of number (aneuploidies) and so far is not amenable to satisfactory medical treatment. However, oral folate is given to all women in the hope of decreasing this condition.

FOR MALE FACTOR

Medical treatment for male infertility is oftentimes difficult and frustrating because even if an identifiable cause is found, immediate results in terms of normal SA are hard to get and persistence with therapy may be required.

i. Endocrine therapy

Infertile males with hypogonadotropic hypogonadism (secondary hypogonadism) are the ones amenable to medical treatments, namely, Gn therapy. For men with hypergonadotropic hypogonadsim (primary testicular failure), there is no evidence that any medical or surgical intervention would help.

ii. Immunologic therapy

Therapy here is with corticosteroids.

iii. Infective therapy

Antibiotics should be given in cases of underlying infection. In fact, oral tetracycline is often given to all males attending most fertility clinics by way of prophylaxis, the drug of choice.

iv. Retrograde ejaculation therapy

Alpha-adrenergic agonists like Tofranil or Sudafed could be used to induce antegrade ejaculation. Otherwise, alkalinization of bladder urine with oral sodium bicarbonate or polycitra could be used prior to sperm retrieval following ejaculation for use in ART.

D. SURGICAL TREATMENTS

FOR THE FEMALE

Advent of modern ART has greatly limited surgeries for female infertility, now mostly limited to few indications as fertility restoration surgeries for the following:

Surgery for ovulation restoration
Laparoscopic ovarian drilling for PCOS

Surgery for tubal occlusive diseases
  Adhesiolysis
  Tubal reversal surgery, including microscopic technique

Surgery for endometriosis
  Adhesiolysis
  Laser ablation

Surgery for uterine anomalies
  Including hysteroscopic resection of submucous fibroids, septate uterus, and bicornuate uterus, etc.

Surgery for other genital structural anomalies
  As seen in such conditions like insertion of Shirodkar's (or McDonald's) suture for cervical incompetence, surgical excision of vaginal septum, etc.

FOR THE MALE

Here, the advent of modern ART actually appears to complement surgeries as these are mostly aimed in either improving sperm quantity and/or quality or aids sperm retrieval from the male reproductive system:

i.   Varicocele ligation
     Varicoceles consist of abnormally dilated testicular veins in the scrotum (pampiniform plexus of veins), most commonly involving the left testicle. They are oftentimes secondary to internal spermatic vein reflux. They are very common findings in the general population, being found in about 15% of all men but even more so in the infertile population (35% of men with primary infertility and 75-81% of those with secondary infertility). Its effect on male fertility is still not very clear as most males with varicoceles are able to father children. A study by Johnson et al. (1970) revealed that 70% of healthy, asymptomatic military recruits with palpable varicoceles had an abnormality on SA. This is further collaborated by a large population study by WHO, 1992, which revealed that varicoceles are accompanied by decreased testicular volume, impaired semen quality, and a decline in Leydig cell function.
     Surgical treatment (varicocele ligation or varicocelectomy) is therefore indicated for those men with abnormal SA or those with other symptoms.

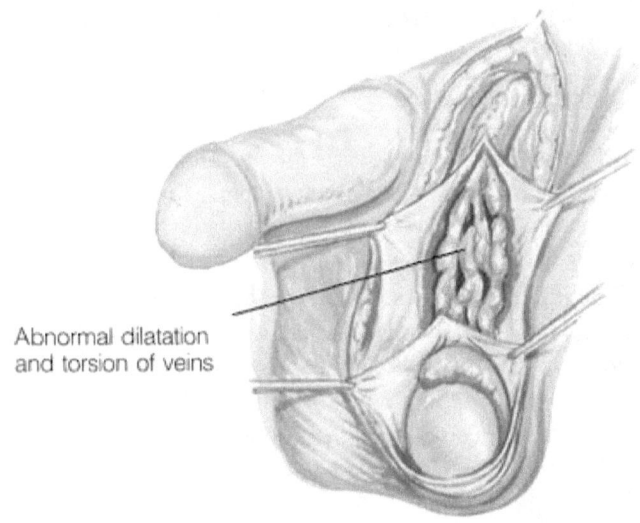

Abnormal dilatation
and torsion of veins

Other studies comparing surgical treatment with nonoperated control groups clearly indicate that varicocelectomy does improve pregnancy rates! (Zini A et al. 1998).

ii.   Sperm retrieval surgeries performed
      Either through the skin
      -   Vasal aspiration with respect to obstruction in the vas and rarely within five years of vasectomy, provides mature sperms equivalent to ejaculated sperms.
      -   Percutaneous epididymal sperm aspiration (PESA)—uses a needle to penetrate the scrotal skin, aiming to draw a small amount of sperm from the epididymis—a blind needle puncture.
      -   Testicular sperm aspiration
      -   Testicular sperm extraction (TESE)—uses a small incision on scrotal skin to remove a small sample of testicular tissue for processing and eventual extraction of sperms.

      Or via microsurgical technique
      -   MicroTESE—an exacting search for sperm under high magnification in cases of extremely low sperm production
      -   Microscopic epididymal sperm aspiration (MESA)

Note that except for vasal aspiration, all the sperm-retrieval procedures provide immature sperms and thus are usually carried out in conjunction with ICSI ART.

E. HIGH-TECH FERTILITY TREATMENTS (High-Tech ART)

These involve achieving fertilization in vitro in a dish with consequent culture in artificial media until ET.

There is usually also a concurrent ovarian hyperstimulation with large quantities of exogenous Gn leading to multiple oocyte development and superovulation.

IN VITRO FERTILIZATION-EMBRYO TRANSFER (IVF-ET)

Treatment of the infertile was based on the traditional concept of identifying and treating causes, but this was largely unsuccessful with respect to infertility treatments until the introduction of IVF-ET in 1978 and its success thereof. There now appears to be a paradigm shift with "skipping over" the causes of infertility when in fact, this procedure was originally conceived to bypass tubal diseases. IVF-ET, colloquially termed test-tube baby, is now being widely and successfully applied in all diverse causes of infertility including "unexplained" infertility and failed IUIs.

In this technique, the egg and the sperms, instead of meeting in the fallopian tube for fertilization to occur, are instead brought together in a dish in the laboratory. After fertilization has occurred, the zygote/s are transferred into the womb to continue growth.

IVF-ET involves a series of process, which, at a glance, could be conceptualized as these ten steps below:

1. Pretreatment

    Usually with BCPs for twenty-one days.

    During this period, all applicable adjunct treatments are commenced—including counseling, lifestyle and dietary changes, acupuncture, multivitamin supplementation (especially folate), and medications such as metformin, prednisone, etc.

2. "Down regulation" of the pituitary gland, depending on chosen protocol

    This involves administering some hormonal treatment to temporarily switch off messages from the brain (hypothalamus) to the ovaries, instructing them to produce and release a matured egg during natural cycles. The fertility specialist then takes over this control function of the brain by now administering other hormones to not only instruct the ovaries to produce matured eggs but even, more importantly, to also manipulate the timing of their release to ensure correct timing for the eggs' retrieval.

3. Stimulation and monitoring of the ovaries for follicle development

    Having now switched off the brain, there is now about two weeks of hormonal treatments to stimulate the ovaries to produce mature eggs such that before natural release, the eggs are collected in a dish. Serial blood hormonal assays and ultrasound measurements are used to monitor success of the treatment. Superovulation is one of the major drawbacks of IVF. It not only dramatically increases costs but it also causes most of the severe complications as well, that is, multiple births and OHSS. Furthermore, it promotes creation of excess embryo, whose management is ethically challenging once created, even within the Catholic doctrine (as there is no dispute that its creation is intrinsically immoral (Donum vitae 1987)).

Occasionally, Gn administration could fail to induce ovarian hyperstimulation and superovulation in some women termed poor or nonresponders. In such cases, a few strategies could be adopted in an attempt to induce ovarian hyperstimulation such as the following:

> even higher dose of Gn (Hofmann GE et al, 1993)
> GnRH flare protocol (Hugues J et al, 1998)
> estrogen pretreatment down regulation (Check JH et al, 1990)
> concomittant GH administration (Homburg R et al, 1991)
> concomittant DHEA administration (Casson PR et al, 2000)

4. Egg retrieval (ER)

As monitoring establishes successful ovarian stimulation, a trigger shot is given for final maturation of the egg/s. About thirty-six hours after the trigger shot, egg retrieval is performed most commonly using a needle, guided by ultrasound through the vagina and to the ovaries. The process only takes a few minutes and often without any anesthesia.

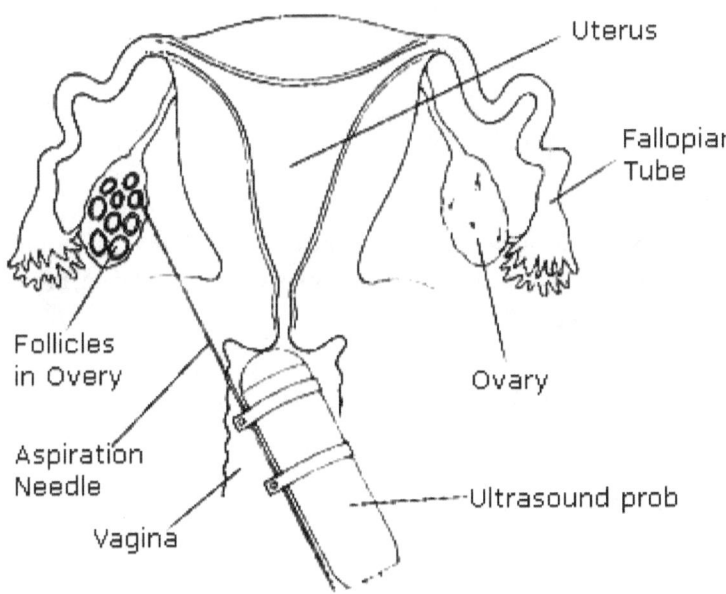

5. Sperm collection and preparation

6. Sperms-eggs incubation (insemination) in a dish in the laboratory for fertilization

   The retrieved eggs are assessed and placed in a dish when a defined number of washed and prepared sperms are added to each egg in a process termed insemination.

7. Early embryo culture

   Following the insemination, the dish is placed in an incubator, and fertilization is assessed after about eighteen hours. The fertilized eggs are now termed embryo, which are further grown in culture for a few days. Below is a microphotograph of a human developing embryo.

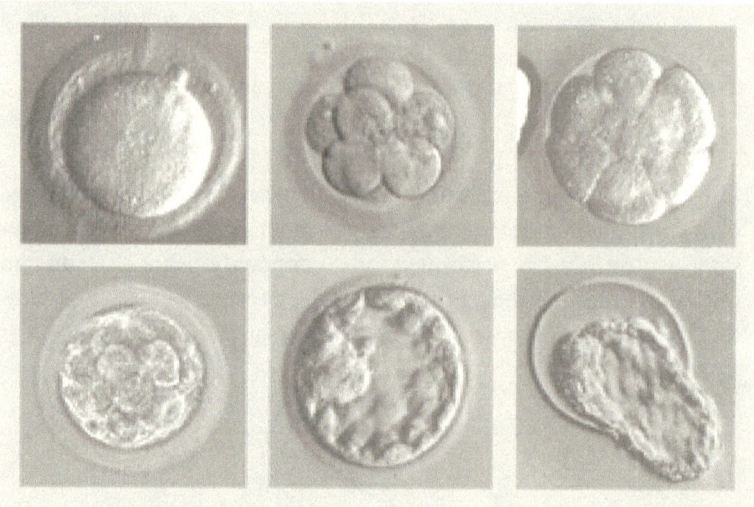

8. ET

   A specified number of embryos are then transferred to the womb with the aid of a narrow plastic tube called the transfer catheter. Again, this takes a few minutes and requires no anesthesia.

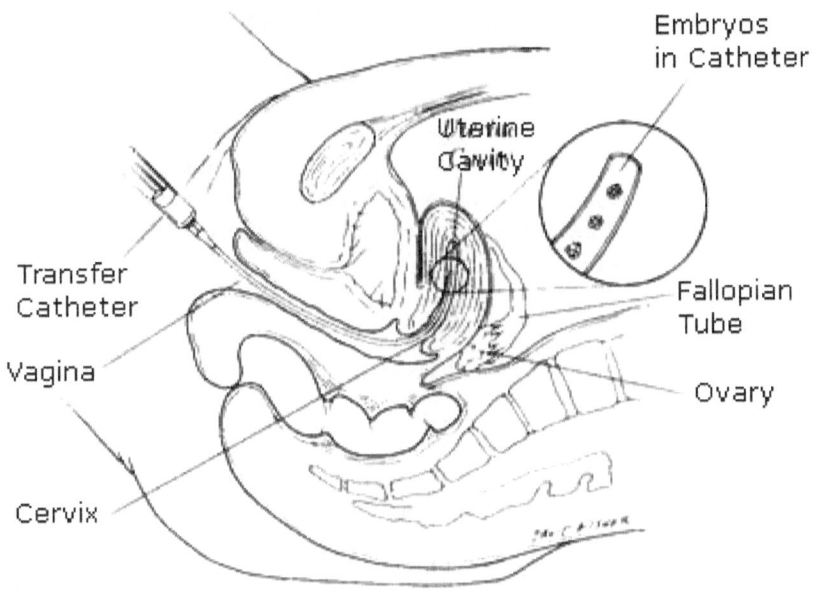

9. Pregnancy confirmation

These are confirmatory tests to establish the success of the treatment cycle, usually performed two to four weeks after ET.

10. Luteal phase support

This is usually employed to hopefully increase the chances of successful implantation. Typically, this involves progesterone administration with or without HCG.

OHSS

Every fertility clinic that undergoes ovarian hyperstimulation/superovulation protocol must also develop a clear management strategy in consonant with the patients to manage OHSS.

OHSS is characterized by significant ovarian enlargement, abdominal pains, bloatedness, nausea, and ascites. The syndrome is usually precipitated by HCG administration, often appearing three to ten days after HCG administration.

Women need to be educated on this potentially serious condition such that once symptom/s appear/s, they should immediately contact the fertility specialist. Strict bed rest with only bathroom privileges and complete avoidance of sexual intercourse or pelvic examination should be instituted. If attendance at other health facilities like the accident/emergency department, the duty physician must be informed of the ovarian hyperstimulation treatment and possible OHSS. Thus, *no pelvic assessment*! All assessment of ovaries must be done by US.

Clinical OHSS has been classified based on clinical symptoms, US findings, and laboratory tests as the following:

1. Mild OHSS

    Here, there are minimal or no symptoms with the ovarian enlargement of less than 6 cm. Management here could be at home with strict bed rest and pelvic rest implemented together with daily monitoring of weight, abdominal girth, and urine output.

2. Moderate OHSS

    Often here, admission to the hospital is indicated with above management plus pain medications.

3. Severe OHSS

    Here, patients have severe abdominal pains, nausea, vomiting, low urine output, shortness of breath, and severe ascites. Admission to the hospital is a must (sometimes into the ICU) with more intensive monitoring, pain medications, and intravenous fluid replacements.

Zygote Intrafallopian Transfer (ZIFT)

This is a high-tech ART different from GIFT in that here, the eggs are inseminated in a laboratory dish to achieve fertilization before transfer to the fallopian tube as per the GIFT procedure.

Micromanipulation ART

i. Intracytoplasmic sperm injection (ICSI)

    This is a highly specialized form of assisted reproductive technology involving microsurgical technique. It was initially developed for severe male infertility, but its indications have increased tremendously for other indications also.

    Here, the steps are essentially the same as for IVF-ET above except for the "high-tech" microsurgical injection of a single sperm directly into the egg to achieve fertilization. Thus, following egg retrieval in the usual manner as in IVF, an initial microsurgical technique is performed to remove the associated cumulus corona radiata complex via repeated passage through fine pipettes as well as treatment with hyaluronidase enzyme to denude the eggs. Only mature eggs in metaphase 2 stage are then used for the definitive microinjection technique to achieve fertilization.

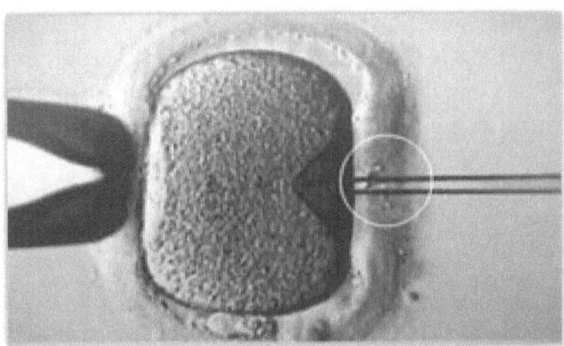

Thereafter, the process continues as per IVF-ET!

ICSI has remained the most effective treatment for male infertility by overcoming the sperm quantity and/or quality problems as the only requirements are for the very few sperms needed to be alive, not necessarily motile and in millions, being only as many sperms as there are eggs to be fertilized! It is thus often performed following prior PESA, MESA, or TESE in the male. The main disadvantages stem from the procedure being very high-tech with more advanced equipment and highly skilled embryologists and hence more costs.

ii. Subzonal sperm injection (SZI)

This micromanipulation ART procedure was developed in the 90's with a fair success whereby a drop of fluid containing sperms is visualized under the microscope from which 5 to 10 healthiest-looking sperms are scooped using a thin hollow glass needle which is also used to penetrate the ZP. The egg and its cell membrane are not penetrated.

iii. Partial zona dissection (PZD)

This is another micromanipulation ART procedure developed by Cohen et al (1990) to assist ZP penetration by sperms. Here micromanipulators are used to pierce the ZP in 2 opposite position. It's use has so far been limited in clinical practice probably with the advent of both ICSI and Assisted Hatching both of which deliver superior advantages with respect to both monospermic fertilization and ZP penetration.

iv. Assisted Hatching (AH)

This is a micromanipulation technique using small pipettes similar to that used for sperm injection although chemicals and even micro-lasers have been used. It is thought to improve implantation although clinically applicable in a few selected patients like in some cases of frozen embryo transfers or older patients or many repeated failed IVF cycles.

v. Preimplantation genetic diagnosis (PGD)

This attempts to diagnose the embryo of any chromosomal anomaly prior to transfer and implantation. There is therefore the suspicion of chromosomal abnormalities as the cause of infertility or recurrent miscarriages.

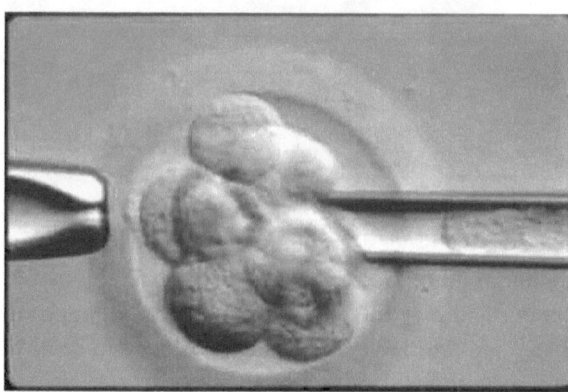

This could be a result of the couple being aware of any existing familial genetic diseases or purely on advancing maternal age or a history of recurrent miscarriages or in certain males with nonobstructive azoospermia.

Unfortunately, it has become one of the most controversial ART, being largely misconstrued by the press as the creation of "designer babies" when in actual fact, it is not possible to manipulate the features or characteristics of an offspring. It is in the realm of science fiction. All PGD achieves is the selection of "healthy" embryos for ET and subsequent implantation.

Donor Egg/Embryo

There are many reasons why donor eggs would be appropriate in certain circumstances like when other ART procedures had been used and failed or when hormonal tests indicate very poor reproductive potential or when the woman has no eggs ab initio, be it absent ovaries at birth or damaged via surgical removal or radiation or chemotherapy, etc.

The first major concern with respect to donor egg procedure is choosing an appropriate donor, either a known donor or from a pool of recruited donors. There is a need for appropriate screenings of potential donors with respect to infectious diseases, genetic and mental health.

Next is counseling for both the donor and the recipient to understand all the ramifications of their decision. It is practical to note that all resulting embryos are owned by the recipient!

Finally, there is the synchronization of the donor with the recipient, such that the egg retrieval (ER) from the donor will match the embryo transfer (ET) in two to three days' time of the recipient's well-prepared and receptive endometrial lining. This is done in a cycle termed coordination cycle with the help of birth control pills (BCP) or GnRH-a (Lupron). Thereafter, while the donor is stimulated to produce mature follicles, the recipient is given estrogen to prepare the endometrium. Once follicular size in the donor reaches 15-18 mm and HCG is being administered in preparation for ER in the donor, progesterone administration is also initiated in the recipient until ET when it is continued as per luteal support. A short course of high-dose prednisone (po prednisone 20 mg od X 3-4 days) is sometimes administered to the recipient starting on the day of ET in the hope of improving outcome and alleviating autoimmunity.

GESTATIONAL SURROGACY

This is also known as the host method. Here, the woman becomes pregnant via ET of a child for which she is not the biological (genetic) mother. This is therefore usually carried out in conjunction with standard IVF, and the mother here is referred to as gestational carrier. This is commonly seen in situations where the woman has no womb or has a medical condition that precludes her from carrying her baby. As such, she is forced to "rent" a womb while using the male partner's semen and genome. Thus, unlike PGD above, the embryo is assumed to be chromosomally normal, but it is the maternal environment that needs to be substituted!

Financial compensation determines altruistic surrogacy or commercial types depending on jurisdiction.

Also, the ethical cum legal issues relating to surrogacy depend on the jurisdiction. There is the popular expectation, albeit in the media, that surrogates feel traumatized after relinquishment of their children, but most studies have not supported such a notion; rather, most surrogates appear to be developing techniques—distancing themselves emotionally from the babies in utero (Terman E, 2003), fostering emotional relationship between the babies and the intended parent (Terman E, 2003), and feeling themselves empowered by the experience (Ragone H, 1994)! India has been at the forefront of commercial surrogacy, which has been legalized since 2002. The state of surrogacy law in Nigeria remains unclear to common folks like me although I suspect that like abortion, it is illegal but still readily available on demand!

F. ADOPTION

This is now increasingly recognized as a reasonable option for individuals or couples who have failed in their desire to achieve their dream family unit. There are, however, many challenges.

Firstly, it is important to realize that adoption per se may not relieve the physical and emotional aspect of infertility, but it could provide the challenges of loving and being loved by the child. Secondly, the costs could be high.

Thirdly, there has been an increasing challenge in finding children for adoption. Even in developed countries, there has been an increasing social acceptance of single parenthood with less and less stigma. The stigma is now instead being slowly directed to brave mothers who dare give up their children for adoption!

Finally, there are, however, numerous legal, cultural, and moral issues and questions to be resolved by the couples such as the following:

- The legal processes involved.
- The type of adoptions available (e.g., open or closed adoption, depending on whether biological and adoptive parents came in contact with one another).
- Use of adoption agencies or available professionals and their specific requirements.
- Are the couple disposed to loving the adopted child as their own?
- What of the other children in the family, extended families, and the society at large?
- Would the adopted child reciprocate love when grown, or would he/she go off to find the birth parents?

Thus, although adoptive parenting may not be the ideal option compared to biological parenting, they are not comparable but very different. It might not be suitable for all individuals and couples unless it is their choice, having made the decision for themselves. Furthermore, although knowledge of adoption as a viable alternative for the management of the infertile abound even in poor developing countries (Oladokun A et al, 2002), cultural biases preclude some from accepting adoption as a viable management option (Araoye MO 2003). Curiously, the Catholic Church promotes adoption in preference to all forms of ART.

G. MEDICAL TOURISM

Medical tourism is a new concept in modern management of infertility. This cross-border medical treatment of disease conditions is already established for certain diseases but growing for infertility treatments worldwide.

Couples even from developed countries seek fertility treatment in a different country for various reasons, but the most common reasons are costs and different regulations/legal frameworks. Data emanating from Europe has shown that a different legal framework is the prime reason for fertility tourism there. For example, the number of eggs that can be fertilized is limited in such countries as Italy while it is the number of embryos to be transferred that is limited in such countries as Germany and the Scandinavian countries; certain procedures like PGD, donor gamete use, surrogacy, or even sex selection is limited in some!

Others reasons for fertility tourism include availability of treatment procedures, wait times for the procedures, and certain cultural characteristics. Also, availability of adverts and full travel arrangements aid to promote certain countries as medical tourism countries. Increased media coverage and the wide availability of Internet services all help to promote medical tourism.

For a developing country like Nigeria, fertility tourism is mostly from Nigeria to developed countries, mostly for the rich few who could afford the treatment. The main reason, however, is unavailability of the procedures. In recent times, there has been an increase in the number of ART units in the countries although these are still quite inadequate and mainly located in a few big cities. Also, a few are now traveling to India instead of the western countries because of lower costs in India.

There are some downsides to fertility tourism such as inadequate follow-up patients and the issue of who manages complications that could arise after such treatments consequent to their return to their own countries. For example, a United Kingdom study found that about one quarter of multiple gestations being cared for in the UK were the results of fertility treatments overseas (McKelvey A et al, 2009)! and this has attendant-costs implication on the home countries' maternity services (Ledger WL et al, 2006).

H. ANCILIARY INFERTILITY TREATMENT

COUNSELING

Counseling should be one of the mainstay of all infertility management, whereby the individuals and couples are provided with opportunity in a confidential environment to explore their thoughts, emotions, reactions, and beliefs with an impartial and sympathetic professional who understands the issues involved.

This is because infertility and its treatment is an extremely stressful condition with both physical and emotional bewilderment for most people who often encounter a mixed bag of intense feelings—namely, anxiety, grief, chronic stress and depression, intense strain on relationships, etc. And all these could be aggravated by modern treatment involving frequent doctor visits and procedures with all the associated costs. Coping strategies should therefore be an important component of infertility treatment. This fact is grossly underemphasized by clinicians in the field. Every couple should be counseled on the coping mechanisms that are even more needed in cases of failed treatment! It is therefore firmly believed that counseling would help maintain good practice with respect to psychosocial health of all patients.

The HFEA *Code of Practice* sets out three frameworks of counseling to be provided for all seeking fertility treatment, namely the following:

1. Implications counseling

    Here, the implications of treatment being proposed will be explored to enable patients/couples understand the implications of the proposed treatments for themselves, their family, and any children born as a result. This is of special significance to those considering surrogacy or using donated sperms, eggs, or embryo, Areas to be dealt with include anonymity, confidentiality, and genetic-risks counseling.

2.   Support counseling

The aim here is to provide emotional support and information at all times but especially in times of particular stress, for example, failure to produce pregnancy or during miscarriage or even high order multiple pregnancy. The hope is to reduce stress by including such strategies as the following:

- Understanding that subfertility is a life crisis, with emotions comparable to the diagnosis of cancer
- Educating them in understanding the basic physiology of reproduction and the poor human female fecundity
- Enabling them to involve a significant other in freely and genuinely communicating their fears, emotions, doubts as well as provide support for each other while understanding differences in coping strategies between different people, different sexes, different races, etc.
- Establishing the "no blame" principle from the outset
- Perhaps even encouraging them to involve other family members and genuine friends in their coping strategies
- Providing access to other couples having similar problems like a form of group-counseling sessions in the clinic
- Encouraging them to pursue other interests
- Encouraging them to have sex during nonfertile periods purely for fun in order to foster closeness and more intimacy in their relationship
- Assuring individuals/couples about utmost respect to their privacy

3.   Therapeutic counseling

Here, expectations are adjusted to the real situations, that is, by recognizing and replacing undesirable or destructive coping mechanisms with constructive coping mechanisms. This is even more applicable in cases of therapeutic failures!

Preconception counseling is a unique form of counseling encompassing elements of the above HFEA framework. Any opportunity that affords young people of childbearing age contact with a health care personnel should ideally be a forum for preconception counseling, be it a young woman seeking advice from a nurse practitioner about contraception and sexual health, a pharmacists dispensing condoms, or a physician treating an STD, etc.

Of special significance is sex education and STD prevention, which should be emphasized at every such opportunity. Optimal health education should be provided, including weight reduction/maintenance strategies, smoking cessation, alcohol and illicit drugs consumption. Smoking has been associated with impaired fertility, spontaneous abortion, ectopic pregnancy, and poor pregnancy outcomes (Stillman RJ, 1989). Illicit drugs such as marijuana has been shown to inhibit GnRH secretion in both males and females and thence affect fertility (Joesoef MR et al, 1993). Even commonly used medications including NSAIDs such as ibuprofen has been shown to block oocyte release, thereby interfering with ovulation (Akil M et al, 1996).

Genetic counseling is a highly specialized field directed at both the couple and their caregivers about genetic risks inherent in achieving their family unit.

Counseling for Catholics

I have consciously added this brief because of my sincere belief as a practicing Catholic that ART does not violate God's law. The background to Catholics doctrinal position (Donum Vitae 1987) is the rejection of nearly all forms of ART as unacceptable, stating that it basically ruptures the unitive and procreative functions of married human sexuality! And two main moral objections are promulgated. First is the ensoulment from conception such that any act (including cryopreservation of embryos aiming to actually preserve the embryo) that might inadvertently endanger the embryo is therefore morally unacceptable. No "spare" embryos may be discarded! The second relates to the nature and purpose of sexual procreation in marriage; that is, human procreation must include a specific act of sexual intercourse, thereby more or less equating sexual intercourse in marriage (conjugal love) as being synonymous with God's love or agape love—the ultimate love. Nowhere is it stated in the Bible that it is immoral for a husband and wife to enjoy sexual relation when they do not intend to procreate! It is unimaginable the kind of love displayed by women and couples seeking ART involving numerous visits to the clinic, numerous transvaginal ultrasounds, numerous injections and pills with their unwanted side effects, including death, not to mention the emotional roller coaster and financial costs. And who could tell a child brought into the world by ART that he or she should not have been brought into existence? As a practicing Catholic myself, I sincerely believe that the principles pronounced in Donum Vitae should guide the use of modern ART for married couples.

ACUPUNCTURE

The use of acupuncture in Western countries has risen dramatically since the 1970s, mainly as an adjunct modality for chronic pain management but now increasingly becoming popular as one of the widely accepted alternative medicine in a variety of other health conditions, including modern infertility treatments. Adjunct traditional Chinese medicine (TCM), especially acupuncture, has been shown in most studies to improve pregnancy outcome for the woman (Magarelli PC et al, 2004) as well as for the men (Gurfinkel E et al, 2003).

The theory behind acupuncture is the claim that it attempts to correct the imbalance in the bioenergy running in the meridian pathways, thereby improving body functions. These bioenergies are further claimed to work via neurotransmitters in nerve endings, especially of the autonomous (sympathetic/parasympathetic) nervous system, which, among others, influence blood flow to organs.

In recent years, a growing number of publications have been appearing in peer-reviewed medical journals. In 2002, Paulus et al. from Germany reported that they had produced a higher clinical pregnancy rate in women undergoing IVF using adjunctive acupuncture compared to those without acupuncture (42.5% v. 26.3%). Since this publication, several other groups have attempted to replicate these results but with conflicting outcomes! This is probably a result of various confounding factors, including the sample populations and statistical analysis used, ovarian stimulation protocol used, type of acupuncture used, etc.

The effectiveness of acupuncture is not solely dependent on the selection of the acupoints but also on the depth of needle insertion as well as the intensity of stimulation. The aim in infertility treatment is often gentle and painless acupuncture administration, which is believed to excite parasympathetic stimulation, thereby increasing blood flow to pelvic organs vis-à-vis sympathetic stimulation following unpleasant, painful, and stressful stimulation that possibly excites alpha-adrenergic receptors!

STRESS REDUCTION

This book is pervaded with the high-stress situation commonly encountered in modern infertility management. As such, and in addition to counseling and acupuncture above, additional active and effective stress reduction strategies should be the norm with all infertility management. These include the following:

- Active relaxation and breathing exercises including adequate sleep and hypnotherapy
- Massage therapy
- Aromatherapy
- Aerobic exercises including yoga
- Faith-based therapy

I. OTHER TREATMENT

ELECTROEJACULATION

By this means, men who, in recent times past, were diagnosed with ejaculatory dysfunction and thence considered infertile because they could not ejaculate, even the presence of spermatozoa production by the testes are now able to be stimulated to induce ejaculation. Subsequently, IUI or other forms of ART could be employed.

Chapter 5

POTENTIAL LOW-COST AND EFFECTIVE ART

There are three kinds of people: those who make things happen;
those who watch things happen and those who wonder how
it happened.

—Anonymous

Successful treatment of infertility with ART, implying IVF, and the methods evolved thereof is now well established although historically, this success has been established without regard to costs of therapy (Ekeh NI, 2008). In fact, ART as is currently being practiced in most developed "resource-rich" countries appears to be further evolving in the high-tech direction as demonstrated by the use of newer, expensive, labor-intensive techniques such as microinjections cum manipulations procedures, including ICSI, AH, PGD.

It has recently been estimated that more than 2 million children have been born worldwide following IVF (Hovatta O et al, 2006). And access to this proven technology, although a worldwide concern, is very miserable for resource-poor countries like Nigeria not only because of cost implications but also because of lack of enabling infrastructures. Otherwise, a state-of-the-art IVF unit could be equipped with reverse-osmosis water-preparation system, advanced air-purification systems, CO_2 incubators, etc., but without infrastructures like constant electricity and water as well as after-sales maintenance capabilities, the unit could potentially end up being a white elephant (Ekeh NI, 2008)!

While 'prevention is always better than cure!', and recognizing the fact that like all disease conditions, it is not always possible to 'prevent' all diseases, infertility inclusive, there is therefore the ongoing need for the proven high-cost, high-tech modern infertility treatment and these should ideally be readily accessible to all, irrespective of the couples financial status or where in the world they are located! Otherwise, there remains a great and urgent need to develop effective, low cost ART alternatives, strategies and modifications (Macklin R, 1995) which could be specially adapted for resource-poor, developing countries although care should be taken not to sacrifice costs at the alter of effective care! As such, the aim should be for a cost-effective care which, by definition, should mandate the ongoing re-engineering of management protocols and equipments dictated by a continuous and a pragmatic search for ever-improving care delivery systems (Gleicher N, 2000).Thus, there is no reason why this could not be by IVF evolving towards simplification and low costs rather than the current tendency for evolution towards more complexity and higher costs.

It is important to briefly outline the major contributor of costs involved in ART, namely the following:

Fixed costs (independent on volume)
> Capital cost (e.g., building costs, equipment costs)
> Overheads (e.g., power, lighting, laundry, cleaning services, some staffing costs)

Variable costs (dependent on volume)
> Medications
> Diagnostic tests
> Consumables, including media
> Some staffing

With respect to ART units, the major cost-consideration areas should uniquely include the following: equipment costs, medications, diagnostic test, consumables, and staffing. And it is in these areas that efforts to establish alternative cheap but effective treatment options (cost-effective management) of infertility should take priority.

1. **Strategies to eliminate or reduce costs associated with Gn therapy**
   These strategies are especially important as a major cost of ART treatment cycle involves the cost of Gn injections to induce superovulation. This is because a major expense for the IVF cycle is the high cost of Gn treatments. Of course, there are other drawbacks of Gn therapy such as the inconvenience of daily injections over a long period of time, side effects of medication of which OHSS is the most significant, and a potentially fatal side effect (Beerendonk CCM et al, 1998). There is also the worrying but unproven risk of ovarian cancer (Whittemore AS, 1994).

   A. Use of natural-cycle IVF
      This involves not using hormones at all and would, of course, be the most economical means of achieving IVF (Hovatta et al. 2006). It is important to recall that the first successful IVF resulting in the

birth of Louise Brown in 1978 was with a natural-cycle IVF. Since no Gn was used, there was also no risk of the potentially life-threatening ovarian hyperstimulation (OHSS) and associated problems of multiple eggs—including multiple pregnancies, unwanted eggs and embryos, etc. There is, however, a major problem with natural-cycle IVF; otherwise, it would not have been abandoned in favor of superovulation. This the need for frequent blood or urine LH assays to monitor egg maturity and then being ready for ER once the egg is matured no matter the time of the day or night. This is a logistic nightmare leading to high cancellation rate, which then makes this approach very unattractive in a modern IVF unit (Ubaldi F et al, 2004)! Some units promoting the concept of natural-cycle IVF use a combination of US natural-cycle monitor and HCG injection to induce ovulation induction as well as timing for ER, all in an attempt to decrease the need for frequent LH assays.

B. Use of inexpensive ovarian stimulation protocols

This commonly employs the use of oral medications such as clomiphene citrate, letrozole, etc., which are much cheaper parenterally than available Gn. Because of the low cost and the ease with which this is combined with IUI in most cases of female infertility involving anovulation (PCOS), this has remained the most widely used ovarian stimulation protocol in modern IVF units, often combining the US monitoring and HCG administration as per above.

C. Mini-IVF with FET

This is a unique approach developed in Japan to simplify IVF and reduce costs. It aims to recruit only a few but high-quality eggs by reducing the number of Gn injections and thence costs as well as risks of OHSS. The protocol is described thus:

Low-dose oral clomiphene citrate is commenced on day 3 and, instead of the usual five days, is continued with follicular tracking to reveal when follicle is mature and due for ovulation. A few booster doses of Gn injections are often administered, usually about three doses on days 8, 10, and 12. Continuing with the clomiphene citrate implies continuing antiestrogenic effects desired centrally on the pituitary where it inhibits the negative feedback of estrogen, making for the release of FSH and also the positive feedback blocking LH release and thence premature ovulation. Ovulation can then be induced when HCG injection is administered. Thus, this cheap, old-fashioned medication popularly called the fertility pill has by this simple change in protocol alleviated the need for pituitary suppression at the beginning of the treatment cycle. However, there is a price to pay as clomiphene citrate also exerts antiestrogen effects peripherally, especially on both the cervical mucus and endometrial linings, often leading hostile cervical mucus to sperms and implantation failures. The effects on cervical mucus are of no consequence here as IVF and even IUI bypass the cervical mucus. However, the Japanese protocol attempts to bypass these peripheral adverse effects by simply freezing the embryos with vitrification as this process has been shown to safely freeze the embryos with virtually no risks of loss. Thereafter, FET can be performed in the next natural cycles.

In the absence of vitrification, some poorly equipped IVF units can attempt add-back estrogen once HCG is administered in the hope that the endometrial lining would be improved, often in conjunction with the standard progesterone luteal phase support.

D. Routine cryopreservation of gametes and embryos with concomitant FET

Poor implantation has continued to be the rate-limiting step in improving pregnancy with ART and, as such, is driving ovarian hyperstimulation with the consequent risks, and harvest of many oocytes and thence more embryos. Embryo cryopreservation, just like sperm cryopreservation, is a well-established routine clinical process with proven success although there are some underlying unique ethical issues. Routine clinical application for human oocyte cryopreservation is still questionable.

The main difference between this and mini-IVF with FET is the fact that gametes (ova and spermatozoa) could also be cryopreserved.

E. Use of in vitro culture and IVM

This is a novel ART technique in which the eggs are retrieved, matured, and fertilized and then transferred (ET), thereby eliminating ovarian hyperstimulation and its attendant time duration, high costs of medications, and 10% risks of OHSS. Thus, unlike conventional IVF where the ovaries are stimulated and the eggs retrieved as close to ovulation as possible, here, the eggs are either not stimulated or just primed with HCG and matured for about twenty-four to forty-eight hours in a medium enriched with some hormones. It is therefore especially applicable to women who have PCOS or at risk for OHSS and occasionally during an IVF cycle when the stimulation protocol allows for many immature eggs to be aspirated as well. The main drawbacks include the fact that it is still a relatively new technique with unclear success rate and long-term outcomes. The immature eggs are very sensitive and prone to damage and loss. Also, there is often a need for ICSI as sperm penetration of the eggs is often problematic.

2. **Strategies to eliminate or reduce costs associated with "high-tech" equipment and maintenance**

A. Timed intercourse

This time-honored, natural family planning approach should more widely be practiced in the management of infertility. However, education and counseling of the couple about the "fertility window" should be at the core for this management option. This is based on the fact that conception can only occur near the time of ovulation. But the exact number of days in the fertile window is not known with certainty as numerous studies give a range of two up to ten! (Bongaarts J, 1983; WHO 1983). Also, a whole lot of other issues are not known for certainty as well such as ideal frequency of intercourse necessary to maximize conception, the timing of intercourse for sex selection (Wilcox AJ et al, 1995).

B. Use of intrauterine insemination (IUI)

This is currently the most widely practiced ART mostly because of its nonreliance on expensive high-tech equipment and expertise. As a routine in most modern IVF clinics, this is often combined with cheap oral ovarian-stimulation protocol, US follicular tracking, and HCG injection to time the IUI. However, the main disadvantage is the exclusion of tubal infertility.

Here, pretreated semen is concentrated in a small volume of 0.2-0.5 ml and injected into the uterine cavity using a catheter. This should be made even more readily available in poor countries as its low cost, ease of technique, and patient friendliness are all reasons why it could be repeated as often as possible until a successful pregnancy is achieved.

C. Use of intravaginal culture (IVC)

This a novel technique that involves incubating the eggs and sperms and even embryos inside the vagina rather than in the CO_2 incubators, which is not only an expensive equipment but is also especially expensive to run and maintain since the environment needs to be such as to nurture the gametes and embryos for an extended period of time.

The principle is based on that of bioencapsulation technology first described by TMS Chang as far back as in 1964! It was later adapted for mammalian reproduction by Nebel et al. (1983). It is only in recent times that a breakthrough with possible clinical applications in humans is being anticipated what with the new field of microfluidics, a science of fluid behavior in a microenvironment (Suh RS et al, 2003), and recent explosive developments in human embryo physiology and metabolism with the attendant difficulties in culture fluids and methods (Torre ML et al, 2007).

In IVC, the gametes (eggs and sperms) are placed in a culture medium in a sterile capsule hermetically sealed and placed inside the woman's vagina, where it is held in place by either a diaphragm or even a tampon. The concept seems very attractive as the woman acts as her own incubator, alleviating the need for the expensive CO_2 incubator as well as maintaining less handling of the gametes and embryos. It has been asserted that if developed, a combination of natural-cycle IVF pus IVC could provide a fertilization rate comparable to conventional IVF and especially be affordable in most resource-poor countries (Hovatta et al. 1996).

Why this concept is still at its infancy is perhaps because of discouragingly low fertilization rates since first been reported by Ranoux et al. in 1988! (Ranoux et al. 1988). Here, they deposited about five harvested oocytes in a tube filled with 3 ml of culture medium and 1 ml of ten to twenty thousand prepared spermatozoa. The tube was then hermetically sealed and placed inside the vagina, held in place by a diaphragm for two to three days and then, cleavage-stage ET undertaken, bypassing expensive CO_2 incubation and sterile culture in a 5% CO_2 enriched environment. Many other studies thereafter reported lower fertilization rates (Costya AL et al, 1991), lower implantation rates even when compared with the more recently introduced day 5 blastocyst ET (Jaroudi K et al, 2004). Yet there is no denying the fact that with the greatly reduced costs, zero risks of OHSS, and no need for expensive CO_2 incubators, this IVC procedure if perfected could be repeated as often as needed to achieve pregnancy, and this may, in fact, in the end lead to comparable pregnancy rate as for conventional IVF! Other patented IVC devices have been studies (Morris R, 2007), but widespread clinical application is still a mirage.

D. Use of intrauterine culture (IUC)

Further extending the concept of IVC is the concept of intrauterine culture cum transfer of gametes (eggs and sperms) for fertilization and implantation in a biodegradable semipermeable capsule, which then acts as temporary incubators, especially for the eggs, which could easily be damaged by direct contact with the endometrium. It is anticipated that by the time of fertilization, the capsule dissolves spontaneously so that the embryo/s could implant. This again has all the advantages of IVC mentioned above but especially less handling of the gametes and embryos such that should this live up to its promise would easily surpass conventional IVF.

IUC would perhaps be the ultimate simplification of all ART if widespread clinical application could be achieved both in terms of logistics, equipment, and costs (Malpani et al. 1991). And yet despite the simplicity of the concept, the clinical application has remained formidable! This is because of the need for cutting-edge technology necessary to manufacture a suitable capsule to be used within the uterine cavity where implantation occurs. It is recognized that despite the tremendous advances in ART in the past twenty-five years or so, with over 75% fertilization rates, implantation rate per embryo transferred has remained the rate-limiting step, at only about 10-15% (Leung CK, 2000). Many reasons have been advocated for this large discrepancy between fertilization rate and implantation rate with ART. Animal studies had already demonstrated that in vivo-produced embryos were less altered compared to in vitro-produced ones, having more intercellular communication devices (Boni R et al, 1999) and more mature mitochondria (Crosier A et al, 2000). Also, it is now well recognized that implantation in vivo is a result of perfect cross talk between a good-quality embryo at the blastocyst stage and a well-prepared, receptive endometrium. Thus, the conventional IVF where ET is routinely performed at cleavage-stage embryo in day 2-3 is presenting an early stage embryo to the endometrium. This is unphysiological and a mismatch ab initio. It is this belief that led to the introduction of extended cultures and cocultures. Simon et al. (1999) demonstrated the beneficial effect of in vitro coculture of the zygote with human endometrial epithelial cells while Barmat et al (1998) did the same with stromal cells. Gardner et al. (1996) utilized a sequential culture system extending cultures to blastocyst stage. And yet all these have not translated into significantly improved implantation rates except for, perhaps, allowing for transfer of embryos with a more proven developmental capacity. Another study (Levran D et al, 2002) attempted to shed some more light on why implantation rate has lagged behind fertilization rate by demonstrating that ZIFT improved outcome in cases of repeated implantation failures with blastocysts possibly raising the notion that perhaps the upper reproductive tract (the fallopian tubes and upper uterus) is probably more beneficial to embryo development and implantation.

All these data support the notion of exploring means of more of in vivo embryo development during ART. One major obstacle why IUC is still at the experimental stage is the difficulty with manufacturing the optimal capsule, which, being a foreign body, might in the end prove detrimental to implantation by not only stimulating uterine contractions but could also elicit endometrial inflammation—a major mechanism of action of commonly available intrauterine contraceptive devices! The disappointing report by Lenz et al. (1991) using biodegradable material and involving twenty-six women with tubal infertility yielded no pregnancy. The major problem encountered in the study was the expulsion of the capsules that were inserted within the endometrial cavity as near the fundus as possible using an insertion tube and piston from an intrauterine device.

In 2001, Dr. Pascal Mock applied for a patent for an intrauterine capsule. This is a retrievable silicon device after five days inside the womb, measuring about 10 mm long and perforated with 360 holes, each measuring about 40 microns to facilitate communication between the embryo and the uterine environment. This device, now called Anecova-d1 device, is being manufactured by a Swiss company, Anecova, created in 2004 by Dr. P. Mock and Martin Velasco.

In October 2009, Anecova proudly announced the safe delivery of the first baby using the device (Blockeel et al. 2009). Anecova is currently pursuing clinical trials in five centers in Europe and Switzerland. This is exciting for ART, especially in developing countries, as Anecova is pledging 10% of its future profits to setting up a foundation to finance projects that will improve ART and their use in developing countries!

Conventional in vitro method   **In Vivo method by Anecova**

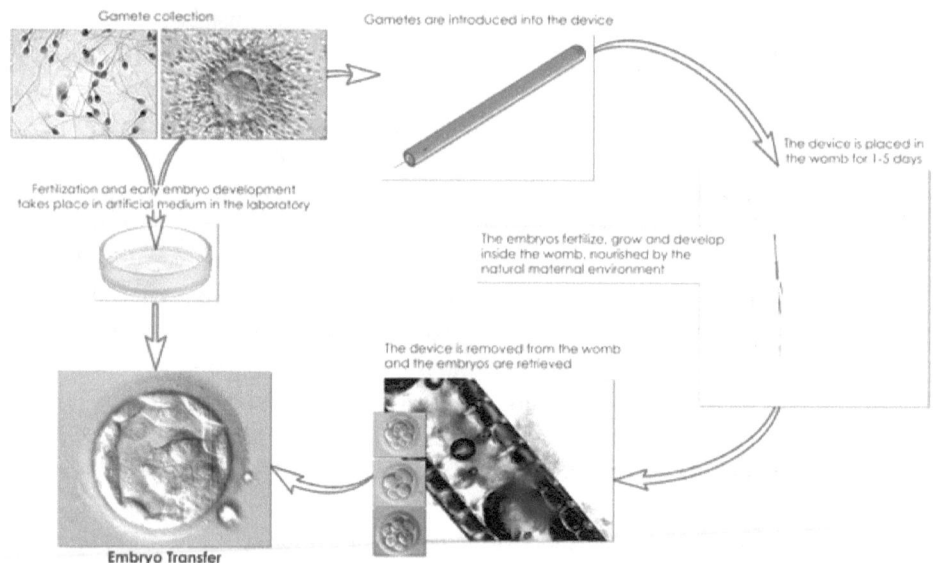

E. Vaginal GIFT

Traditional GIFT via laparoscopy has most of the advantages of IVC and IUC, including less handling of gametes/embryos and no need to invest in expensive CO_2 incubators, but it still has the major disadvantage of requiring laparoscopy for the gamete transfer. (See GIFT, chapter 4.) Hence, the attempt to develop vaginal GIFT by Jansen et al. (1987), who recently devised special catheter sets that could allow the gametes to be introduced into the fallopian tubes under US guidance. Pregnancy rate with GIFT should ideally be greater than that of conventional IVF as fertilization and nurturing of the embryo is occurring in vivo inside the fallopian tube where they "belong" with its physiological milieu rather than a dish in the laboratory. Of course, it is pertinent to note that this technique is officially sanctioned by the Roman Catholic Church with some provisos such as the procedure being carried out on a married couple following sexual intercourse without allowing in vitro contact between the gametes and no attempt at fetal reduction of possible excess conceptions, etc!

F.   Fallopian tube sperm perfusion (FSP) (Trout SW et al, 1999)

This is an attempt to overcome the perceived limitations of IUI by ensuring more spermatozoa reaching the fallopian tubes at the time of ovulation. This is because studies of the dynamics of sperm transport have shown a progressive decline in the number of sperms along the length of the female reproductive tract such that in normal fallopian tubes, a maximum of only two hundred spermatozoa are present in male subfertility (Fishel et al. 1982). Kahn et al (1992) was the first to report the clinical experience with FSP using the Frydman catheter while Li TC (1993) described a simple technique of FSP, whereby a pediatric Foley's catheter is used to infuse a large sperm volume (4 ml) into the uterine cavity with the inflated balloon positioned at the internal cervical os to prevent fluid reflux. Another variant uses a specially adapted device called sperm perfusion device (Fanchin R et al, 1995). With this large volume, spermatozoa not only perfuse the fallopian tubes but also spill into the pouch of Douglas. However, the jury is still out there with respect to differences in pregnancy rates between standard IUI and FSP.

G.   Transport IVF/ICSI

A good IVF unit needs a high-tech laboratory with standards, high-tech equipment, and expertise to be able to maintain the eggs, sperms, and embryos in an optimal environment in the laboratory. This has been a major limiting factor in the establishment of IVF units, especially in resource-poor countries. It could therefore be possible, even for the government of third world countries, to set up one such standard IVF laboratory such that ER could be carried out in peripheral units and hospitals, transported in its follicular fluids in a specially designed incubator to the central laboratory where the eggs are "processed." The incubator could be plugged unto the car battery or that of airplanes. In the few countries where this is in practice at the present, all IVF laboratory procedures, and later the ET, are all carried out in the central laboratory. The advantages of this method include the need to establish only very few high-quality laboratories and concentrated staff with expertise and the "numbers" to maintain the high standards and high pregnancy rates. Also, this encourages the involvement of a local gynecologist to care for their patients as they perform the ERs in their peripheral clinics/hospitals.

H. Use of commercial culture media

It is important to realize that until recently, most IVF laboratories manufacture their own culture media with very expensive equipment and the need for scrupulous testing and quality control to ensure that each batch is toxin free and can maintain embryo growth. However, and in recent times, there are many commercially available culture media that can be bought off the shelf, which has helped in greatly reducing the costs of establishing and running modern IVF laboratories and, in addition, minimizing one of the variables inherent in "in-house" culture media by each laboratory, which leads to variable pregnancy rates!

3. Others
   -   Adjunctive use of acupuncture to improve pregnancy outcome

Chapter 6

WHEN EVERYTHING SEEMS TO FAIL

God, grant me the serenity to accept the things I cannot change, the courage to change the things I can change, and the wisdom to know the difference.

—Rainhold Niebuhr

Rachel asked her maid to give her children by Jacob.

—Genesis 30

The continuing attempt at domination of scientific manipulation of nature has created an apparent illusion that we can now scientifically control procreation with modern contraception and ART. Thus, one of the most difficult problems in modern infertility management is deciding when enough is enough! This is with respect to not only the couples but also the physician. The ability to continue more attempts at treatment, coupled with evolving newer technologies, gives the treating physicians more optimism that with further treatments, the couples will eventually get pregnant while the couples themselves are conditioned with the notion that if they try hard enough and persevere, they would get pregnant. And with the pace of advances in modern infertility management, there is never a lack of new advances and thence new avenues of hope especially for the infertile couple!

Therefore, there is always the need when everything seems to fail for a suitable opportunity to reevaluate various options between the treating physicians and the couple, especially those not already pursued in the course of infertility management per se.

- Using donor sperms or eggs
- Surrogacy
- Adoption
- Fostering
- Remaining childless

All these above could provide a viable alternative to accomplish your ideal family unit except the last which implies that the couple have resigned themselves to life with out the desired family unit or even child-free life. Again this may not be an easy decision, bearing in mind that either of the couple or the treating physician might be at different stage of acceptance of the perceived failures to achieve the couple's ideal family unit. Also and especially in developing countries with poor social support, one of the biggest fears about opting for a child-free life is the fear of regret later in old age with no children to look after one self. This is unlike the developed countries where social services and support could provide care for the poor and aged. On the other hand, since raising children could be an expensive project, it could be argued that the infertile without a child to raise could potentially be saving to off-set the costs needed in old age.

There is also the need for emotional support and counselling as a number of studies seem to suggest that some of the most stressful situations regarding infertility and its treatment is not the medical procedures per se but the fact of trying to become pregnant with or without ART and not succeeding! (Baram et al, 1988; Connoly et al, 1993; Boivin et al, 1995; Leiblum et al, 1998).

Even the Catholic Church's opposition to all forms of modern ART basically offers the bottom line position here for infertile couple to remain childless, and more or less wait on GOD for a miracle!

Finally, there have been many anecdotal reports of spontaneous pregnancies after failed treatments even with expensive high tech ART, perhaps a miracle from GOD.

Appendices

Glossary

ART (assisted reproductive technology)

This includes any treatment or procedure involving the handling of eggs and sperms in order to establish pregnancy such as IUI, GIFT, ZIFT, IVF-ET, ICSI, embryo cryopreservation, egg/embryo donation, surrogacy, etc.

ART cycle

This is a timed sequential processes involving ART. It usually commences with intake of fertility drugs and/or cycle monitoring.

blastocyst

The implantation stage spherical cell mass (five to seven days old embryo with 50-150 cells) formed from the morula and consisting of an outer layer of cells (the trophectoderm), a fluid-filled cavity (the blastocoel), and the inner cell mass.

donor embryo/gamete (egg or sperm)

This involves use of another person's gametes or embryo in a substitute unable to produce own gametes or embryos termed the recipient.

conception

Fertilization following successful union of the egg and sperm.

copulation

Act of sexual intercourse.

egg

This is the female reproductive cell, also termed ovum or oocyte.

ejaculation

Sudden and forceful ejection of semen (usually containing sperms) accompanying orgasm from the male reproductive system in the final stages of sexual intercourse.

embryo

The developing organism from the time of fertilization until the formation of organs at the end of the eighth week of gestation when the organism is generally termed a fetus.

emission

Involuntary discharge of semen, say, during sleep.

epidemiology

A branch of medicine that tries to define the causes, prevalence, and control of diseases in a defined population.

exocytosis

A process of secretion or excretion by cells, whereby chemical substances in vesicles within the cell are discharged from the cell via fusion between the vesicular membrane and the cell membrane.

fecundity

The capacity of female organisms to reproduce rapidly and in great numbers.

fertilization

The penetration of an egg by the sperm and subsequent fusion of their genetic material to form an embryo.

fetus

An unborn child from about eight weeks' intrauterine life with recognizable features and until birth.

follicle

This is a structure within the ovaries that contain an egg.

gamete

This is reproductive cell, either an egg or a sperm.

hormones

A chemical substance produced to control and regulate the activities of certain cells or organs. It could act locally or in a distant organ being transported by the blood.

implantation

Embedded. In embryology, this refers to the attachment of the developing embryo into the uterine cavity, usually at the blastocyst stage on days 5-7 postconception.

laparoscopy
> A minimally invasive surgical procedure in which a fiber optic instrument termed laparoscope is inserted via the abdominal wall to visualize pelvic structures

menstruation
> The periodic shedding of uterine lining in a woman of reproductive age when conception fails to occur.

morula
> A solid mass of cells termed blastomeres and formed as the zygote splits up to the sixty-fourth cell stage.

ovulation
> The discharge of a mature egg from the ovary.

paracrine
> Para = alongside; near; next to.
> Relates to the release of chemical substances or hormones into adjacent cells or tissues rather than distant tissues via the bloodstream.

pre-embryo
> This is a fertilized egg in the early stages of development prior to cell division.

pregnancy
> This could be biochemical based on detection of HCG in the urine or blood, or clinical based on the detection of gestational sac on ultrasound.

reproduction
> One of the biological characteristics of living things that enables generation of identical offspring.

semen
> The thick white fluid containing sperms that is ejaculated by the male reproductive tract.

sperm
> The male reproductive cell.

spermatogenesis
> The process of sperm production in the testes.

spermiogenesis

> The final stage of spermatogenesis, whereby the spermatids mature into the motile spermatozoa or sperms.

trophectoderm

> The cells forming the outer layer of the blastocyst that differentiates into the trophoblast and thence the placenta.

zygote

> The cell (now diploid) that results from the union of the male and female gametes at fertilization.

Bibliography

Abdelkader AB, Yeh J. The potential use of intrauterine insemination as a basic option for infertility: A review for Technology-limited medical settings. http://www.hindawi.com/journals/ogi/2009/584837.html

Akil M, Amos RS, Stewart P. Infertility may sometimes be associated with NSAID consumption. Br J Rheumatol 1996; 35: 76-8

Araoye MO. Epidemiology of infertility; social problems of the infertile couples. W Afr J Med 2003; 22(2): 190-6

Baram D, Tourtelot E, Muechler E, Huang K. Psychosocial adjustment following unsuccessful in vitro fertilization. J Psychosom Obstet Gynaecol 1988; 9: 181-90.

Barmat LI, Liu HC, Spandoefer SD, Xu K, Veeck L, Damario MA, Rosenwaks Z. Human preembryo development on autologous endometrial coculture versus conventional medium. Fertil Steril 1998; 70: 1109-13.

Barnhart K, OsheroffJ. We are over interpreting the predictive value of serum FSH levels. Fertil Steril 1999; 72: 8-9.

Bartoov B, Eltes F, Pansky M et al. Improved diagnosis of male fertility potential via a combination of quantitative ultramorphology and routine semen analysis. Hm Reprod 1994; 9: 2069-74.

Basso O, Weinberg CR, Baird DD, Wicox AJ, Olsen J. Subfecundity as a correlate of preeclampsia; a stuy within the Dannish National Birth Cohort. Am J Epidemiol 2003; 157(3): 195-202

Basso O, Olsen J. Subfercundity and neonatal mortality; Longitudinal study within the Dannish National Birth Cohort. BMJ 2005; 330(7488): 393-4.

Beerendonk CCM, van Dop PA, Merkus JMWM. Ovarian hyperstimulation syndrome: facts and fiction. Obstet Gynecol Surv 1998; 53: 439-49.

Berkovitz A, Eltes F, Soffer Y et al. ART success and in vivo sperm selection depend on the ultramorpholoical status of spermatozoa. Andrology 1999; 31: 1-8

Bischof P, Meisser A, Campana A. Paracrine and autocrine regulators of trophoblast invasion-a review. Placenta 2000; 21(A): S55-S60.

Blockeel C, Mock P, Verheyen G, Bouche N, Le Goff Ph, Heyman Y, Wrenzycki C, Hoffmann K, Niemann H, Haentjens P, de Los Santos MJ, Fernandez-Sanchez M, Valesco P, Aebischer P, Deveroey P, Simon C. An in vivo culture system for human embryos using an encapsulation technology: a pilot study. Human Reprod 2009; 1(1): 1-7

Boerma JT, Urassa M. Association between infertility, HIV and sexual behaviour in rural Tanzania. In Boerma JT & Urassa M (eds). Women and Infertility in sub-Sahara Africa: A multi-disciplinary perspective 2001, Royal Tropical Institute, Amsterdam: 179-85.

Boivin VJ, Hennessey JF. Emotional aspects and support in in vitro fertilization and embryo transfer program, J In Vitro Fertil Embryo Transfer 1988; 5: 290-5.

Bongaarts J. The proximate determinants of natural marital fertility. In: Determinants of fertility in developing countries. Eds; Bulatao RA, Lee RD, Hollerbach PE, Bongaarts J. New York, Academic Press 1983: 103-38.

Boni R, Tosti E, Roviello S, Dale B. Intracelular communication in in vivo and in vitro produced bovine embryos. Biol Reprod 1999; 61: 1050-5.

Boomsma CM, Heineman MJ, Cohlen BJ, Farquhar C. Semen Preparation techniques for intrauterine insemination. The Cochrane Database of systematic reviews 2007; 4: 1-29

Casson PR, Lindsay MS, Pisarska MD, Carson SA, Buster JE. Dehydroepiandrosterone supplementation augments ovarian stimulation in poor responders: a case series. Hum Reprod 2000; 15(10): 2129-32.

Cates W, Farely TMM, Rowe PJ. Worldwide patterns of infertility: is Africa different? The Lancet 1985; 2(8455): 596-8

Chang TMS. Semipermeable microcapsules. Science 1964; 164: 524-5

Check JH, Nowroozi K, Chase JS et al. Ovulation induction and pregnancies in 100 consecutive women with hypergonadotrophic amenorrhoea. Fertil Steril 1990; 70: 107-10

Connolly KJ, Edelman RJ, Cooke ID, Robson J. The impact of infertility on psychological functioning. J Psychosom Res 1992; 36: 459-68

Congregation for the Doctrine of the Faith, Instruction on respect for human life in its origin and the dignity of procreation (Donum Vitae). San Francisco; Ignatius Press 1987: intro 4.

Cooke ID. Failure of implantation and its relevance to subfertility. J Reprod Fertil Suppl 1988; 36: 155-9.

Costoya AL, Cafatti CM, Gadan A. Experience with intravaginal culture for in vitro fertilization. J Assist Reprod Gen 1991; 8(6): 360-1

Coutifaris C, Myers ER, Guzick DS, McGovern PG, Schlaff WD et al. Histological dating of timed endometrial biopsy tissue ie not related to fertility status. Fertil Steril 2004; 82(5): 1264-72.

Creus M, Panarraubia J, Fabreques F, Vidal E, Carmonia F, Casamitjana R, Vandrell JA, Balasch J. Day 3 serum inhibin B, FSH and age as predictors of assisted reproductive treatment outcome. Hum Reprod 2000; 15: 2341-6

De Vet A, Laven JS et al. a putative marker for ovarian aging. Fertil Steril 2002; 77: 357-62

Donum Vitae. Instruction on Respect for Human Life in its Origin and on the Dignity of procreation; Congregation of doctrine of the faith, 1987.

Ekeh NI. Comparing the cost and cost-effectiveness of standard IVF therapy with alterative, novel, low-cost ART treatment techniques namely: Intra Vaginal Incubation and Embryo transfer (IVC + ET); Intra Uterine Culture.

Evers JL, Slaats P, Land JA et al. Elevated levels of basal estradiol 17 Beta predict poor response in patients with normal basal level of FSH undergoing in vitro fertilization. Fertil Steril 1998; 69:1010-4.

Fanchin R, Olivennes F, Hazout A, Frydman R. Anew system for fallopian tube sperm perfusion leads to pregnancy twice as high as standard intrauterine insemination. Fertil Steril 1995; 64: 505.

Franklin S. Embodied Progress: A cultural account of Assisted Conception. Routledge 1997: London, New York

Fishel SB, Edwards RG. Essentials of fertilization. In: Human conception In Vitro; Eds: Edwards RG, Purdy JM. Academic Press, London 1982; 157-79

Gardner DK, Lane M, Calderone I, Leeton J. Environment of the preimplantation human embryo in vivo: metabolite analysis of oviduct and uterine fluids and metabolism of cumulus cells. Fertil Steril 1996; 65: 349-53

Gates W, Farley TMM, Rowe PJ. Worldwide patterns of infertility: Is Africa different? Lancet 1985; 2: 596-8

Gleicher N. Cost-effective infertility care. Hum Reprod Update 2000; 6(2): 190-9

Greenhall E, Vessey > The prevalence of subfertility: a review of the current confusion and a report of two new studies. Fertil Steril 1990; 54(6): 978-83.

Gurfinkel E et al. Effects of acupuncture and moxa treatment in patients semen abnormalities. Asian J Androl 2003; 5(4): 345-8.

Guzick DS, Carson SA, Coutifaris C et al. "Efficacy of superovulation and intrauterine insemination in the treatment of infertility'. New Eng J Med 1999; 340(3): 177-83.

Hotaling JM, Walsh TJ. Male infertility: a risk factor for testicular cancer. Nature Reviews Urology 2009; 6: 550-6.

Hofmann GE, Toner JP, Muasher SJ et al. High-dose FSH ovarian stimulation in low responder patients for in vitro fertilizayion. J In Vitro Fert Embryo Trans 1993; 6: 285-9

Homburg R, Eshel A, Abdulla HI et al. Growth hormone facilitates ovulation induction by gonadotrophins. Clin Endocrinol 1988; 29: 113-5.

Hovatta O, Cooke I. Cost-effective approaches to in vitro fertilization: Means to improve access. Int J Obstet Gynecol 2006; 94: 287-91

Hugues J, Durnerin I. Revisiting gonadotrophin-releasing hormone agonist protocols and management of poor ovarian responses to gonadotrophins. Hum Reprod Update 1998; 4: 83-101.

Hull MGR, Glazener CMA, Kelly NJ et al. Population study of causes, treatment and outcome of infertility. BMJ 1985; 291: 1693-7.

Ibe IN, et al. Dietary exposure to aflatoxin in human male infertility in Benin City, Nigeria. Int J Fertil 1994; 39(4): 208-14.

Jansen RPS, Anderson JC. Catheterisation of the fallopian tubes from the vagina. Lancet 1987; 2: 366

Jaroudi K, Al-Hassan S, Sieck U, Al-sufyan H, Al-Kabra M, Coskun S. Zygote transfer on day 1 versus cleavage stage embryo transfer on day 3: a prospective trial. Hum Reprod 2004; 19(3): 645-8

Jayaprakasan K, Campbell BK, Clewes IR, Raine-Fenning NJ. Three-dimensional ultrasound improves interobserver reliability of antral follicle counts and facilitates increased clinical work flow. Ultrasound Obstet Gynecol 2008; 31: 439-44

Joesoef MR, Beral V, Aral SO, Rolfs RT, Cramer DW. Fertility and use of cigarettes, alcohol, marijuana, and cocaine. Ann Epidemiol 1993; 3(6): 592-4

Joffe M, Li Z. Association of time of pregnancy and the outcome of pregnancy. Fertil Steril 1994; 62(1): 71-5.

Kahn JA, von During V, Sunde A, Sordal T, Molne K. Fallopian tube sperm perfusion. First clinical experience. Hum Reprod 1992; 7: 19-24

Kosmas IP, Tatsioni A, Fatemi HM, Kolibianakis EM, Tournaye H, Devroy P. Human chorionic gonadotrophin administration vs luteinizing hormone monitoring for intrauterine insemination timing, after administration of clomiphene citrate: a meta analysis. Fertil Steril 2007; 87(3): 607-12.

Kruger TF, Swanson RJ, Acosta AA et al. Predictive value of anormal sperm morphology in in vitro fertilization. Fertil Steril 1988; 49: 112-17

Kuku SF, Osegbe DN. Oligozoospermia in Nigeria. Archives of Andrology 1989; 22: 233-8.

Lalich RA, Marut EL, Prins GS et al. Life table analysis of intrauterine insemination pregnancy rates. Am J Obstet Gynecol 1986; 4: 824-980.

Lass A, Skull J, Mc Veigh E, Margara R, Winston RM. Measurement of ovarian volume by transvaginal sonography before ovulation induction with human menopausal gonadotrophin for in itro fertilization can predict poor response. Hum Reprod 1997; 12: 294-7.

Ledger WL, Anumba D, Marlow N, Thomas CM, Wilson EC. Cost of Multiple Births Study Group (COMBS Group). The costs to the NHS of multiple births after IVF treatment in the UK. BJOG 2006; 113: 21-5.

Leiblum SR, Aviv A, Hamer R. Life after infertility treatment: a long-term investigation of marital and sexual function. Hum Reprod 1998; 13: 3569-74

Leung CK. Recent advances in clinical aspects of in vitro fertilization. Hong Kong Med J 2000; 62: 169-76

Levran D, Farhi J, Nahum H, Royburt M, Glezerman M, Weissman A. Prospective evaluation of blastocyst stage transfer vs zygote intrafallopian tube transfer in patients with repeated implantation failure. Fertil Steril 2002; 77: 971-7

Li TC. A simple, non-invasive method of fallopian tubes sperm perfusion. Hum Reprod 1993; 8: 1848-50

Lunenfield B, Van Steireghem A. Infertility in the third millennium: Implications for the individual, family and society. Condensed meeting report from the second Bartarelli Foundation's global conference. Hum Reprod Update 2004; 10(4): 10

Macklin R. Reproductive technologies in developing countries. Bioethics 1995; 9: 276-82

Magarelli PC et al. Acupuncture and good pronosis IVF patients: Synergy. Fertil Steril 2004; 84: 20.

Malpani A, Malpani A Simplifying assisted conception techniques to make them universally available-a view from India. Hum Reprod 1991; 7: 49

Mashiach R, Fisch B, Eltes F et al. The relationship between sperm ultrastructural features and fertilizing capacity in vitro. Fertil Steril 1992; 57: 1052-57.

McKelvey A, David A, Shenfield F, Jauniaux ER. The impact of cross-border reproductive care or 'fertility tourism' on NHS maternity services. BJOG 2009; 116: 1520-3.

Morris RL. Assessment of Efficacy and Acceptability of a new device used to incubate gametes during Intravaginal culture. In: http??www.ivfl.com. 2007.

Nahim R, Shifren JL, Chang Y, Leykin L, Isaacson K, Toth TI. Antral follicle assessment as a tool for predicting outcome in IVF-Is it better predictor than age and FSH? J Assist Reprod Henet 2001; 18: 15105.

Nebel RL, Bame JH, Saackie RG, Lim F. Microencapsulation of bovine spermatozoa. I Anim Sci 1983; 60(6): 1631-9

NICE Guidelines. National Institute for Clinical Excellence, Fertility: Assessment and treatment of people with fertility problems, RCOG Press 2004; London, UK.

Okonofua FE. The case against new reproductive technologies in developing countries. BJOG 1996; 103: 957-62.

Okonofua F. Infertility and woman's reproductive health in Africa. Afri J Reprod Health 1999; 3(1): 7-9

Okonofua F. New Reproductive Technologies and infertility treatment in Africa. Afri J Reprod Health 2003; 7(1): 7-8

Oladokun A, Arulogun OS, Oladokun R, Morhason-Bello O, Bamgboye E, Adewole I, Ojengbede O. J Obstet Gynecol 2002; 22(2): 211-6

Osuna C, Matorras R, Pijoan JI, Rodriguez-Escudero FJ. One versus two inseminations per cycle in intrauterine insemination with sperm from patients' husbands: a systematic review of literature. Fertil Steril 2004; 82(1): 17-24

Parnell T. Systematic review on the prevalence and epidemiology of infertility 1999-2004. (Study Protocol). Training in Reprod Health Res, Gen 2005.

Paulus WE, Zhang M, Strehler E, El-Danasouri I, Sterzik K. Influence of acupuncture on the pregnancy rate in patients who undergo assisted reproduction therapy. Fertil Steril 2002; 77(4): 721-4.

Population Report Series 1, 1983; 11(3)

Ragone H. Surrogate Motherhood: Conception in the heart. Westview Books 1994.

Reproductive Health Outlook. Infertility: Overview/lessons learned 1997-2005. http://www.rho.org

Schmidt L, Munster K, Helm P. Infertility and the seeking of infertility treatment in a representative population, Br J Obstet Gynecol 1995; 102: 978-84.

Seifer DB, Maclaughlin DT et al. Early follicular serum Mullerian-inhibiting substance levels are associated with ovarian response during assisted reproductive technology cycles. Fertil Steril 2002; 77: 468-71

Seifer DB, Scott RJ Jr et al. Women with declining ovarian reserve may demonstrate a decrease in day 3 inhibin B before a rise in day 3 FSH. Fertil Steril 1999; 72: 65-7.

Simon C, Mercader A, Garcia-Velasco J, Nikas G, Moreno C, Remohi J, Pellicer A. Coculture of human embryos with autologous human endometrial epithelial cells in patients with implantation failure. J Clin Endocrinol Metab 1999; 84: 2638-48.

Smotrich DB, Widra EA, Gindoff PR et al. Prognostic value of day 3 estradiol on in vitro fertilization outcome. Fertil Steril 1995; 64: 1136-40

Steptoe PC, Edwards RG. Birth after the manipulation of a human embryo. Lancet 1978; 2: 366

Stillman RJ. Smoking and reproductive health. Semin Reprod Endocrinol 1989; 7: 291-348.

Teman E. 'The Medicalization of Nature' in the Artificial Body: Surrogate motherhood International in Israel. Medical Anthropology Quarterly 2003; 17(1): 78-98

Teman E. Knowing the surrogate body in Israel In: Rachel Cook and Shelley Day (eds) Surrogate motherhood; International Perspective, London. Hart Press pp 261-80

te Velde ER, Parson PL. The variability of female reproductie aging. Hum Reprod Update 2002; 8: 141-54

Tiettze C. Reproductive span and rate of conception among Hetterite women. Fertil Steril 1957; 8: 89-97.

Tomas C, Nuojua-Huttunen S, Martikainen H. Pretreatment transvaginal ultrasound examination predicts ovarian response to gonadotrophins in in-vitro fertilization. Hum Reprod 1997: 12: 220-3.

Torre ML, Faustini M, Attilio KME, Vigo D. Cell Encapsulation in Mammal Reproduction. Recent Patent on Drug Delivery & Formulation 2007; 1: 81-5

Trou SW, Kemman E. Fallopian tube sperm perfusion versus intrauterine insemination: a randomized controlled trial and metaanalysis of the literature. Fertil Steril 1999; 71: 881-5

Ubaldi F, Rienzi L, Ferrero S et al. National in vitro fertilization cycles. Annals of the New York Academy of Sciences 2004; 1034: 245-51

van Noord-Zaastra BM, Looman CW, Asbach H, Habbema JD, te Velde ER, Karbaat J. Delaying childbearing: effect of age on fecundity, and outcome of pregnancy. BMJ 1991; 302: 1361-5.

Van Rooij IA, Broekman FJ et al. Serum anti mullerian hormone levels: a novel measure of ovarian reserve. Hum Reprod 2002; 17: 3065-71

Wallace WHB, Kelsey TW. Human Ovarian Reserve from conception to the menopause. PLoS ONE 2010; 5(1): e8772.10.1371/journal.pone.0008772.

Warburton D, Kline J, Stein Z, Cytogenetic abnormalities in spontaneous abortion of recognized conception. In: Porter IH, editor. Perinatal genetics: Diagnosis and treatment. NY: Academic Press 1986; p 133.

Weghofer A, Feichtinger W. The forgotten variable impact of luteinizing hormone on the prediction of ovarian reserve. Fertil Steril 2006; 85: 259-61

Whittemore AS. The risk of ovarian cancer after treatment for infertility. N Engl J Med 1994; 331: 805-6.

WHO (1991). Infertility. A tabulation of available data on prevalence of primary and secondary infertility. Geneva. Programme on Maternal and Child Health and Family Planning Division of Family Health, WHO, 1991.

WHO (1992). The influence of varicocele on parameters of fertility in a large group of men presenting to infertility clinics. Fertil Steril 1992; 57:1289.

WHO (2002). Vayena E, Rowe P, David Griffin P (editors). In Introduction: Current Practices and Controversies in Assisted Reproduction 'Medical, Ethical and Social Aspects of Assisted Reproduction' Geneva: WHO 2002; 15-7.

WHO (2010) WHO Laboratory Manual for the examination and processing of human semen. Fifth Edition

Wilcox AJ, Weinberg CR, Baird DD. Timing of intercourse in relation to ovulation-Effects on the probability of conception, survival of the pregnancy, and sex of the baby. N Engl J Med 1995; 333: 1517-21.

Wilcox AJ, Baird DD, Weinberg CR. Time of implantation of the conceptus and loss of pregnancy. N Engl J Med 1999; 340(23): 1796-9.

Zini A, Buckspan M, Berardinucci D et al. Loss of left testicular volume in men with clinical left varicocele: correlation with grade of varicocele. Arch androl 1998; 41: 37:

Index

W

WHO (World Health Organization), xx, 1-2, 7

Z

Zygote Intrafallopian Transfer (ZIFT), 48, 63

www.ingramcontent.com/pod-product-compliance
Lightning Source LLC
Chambersburg PA
CBHW022100170526
45157CB00004B/1413